EXERCISES FOR SENIORS OVER 60

LYDIA STRETCH

TABLE OF CONTENTS

Introduction:

Embracing Movement, Enhancing Life

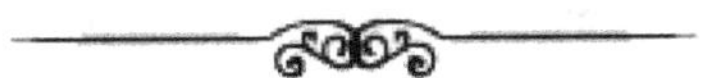

Welcome to a journey designed to empower, uplift, and energize you. This book is about celebrating what your body can do, exploring how movement can improve every aspect of your life, and finding joy in the steps, stretches, and small victories along the way. Whether you're just starting to explore fitness or looking to build on what you've already accomplished, this guide will be with you each step, reminding you that every bit of effort brings rewards—not just in health but in how you feel every day.

Exercise is one of the most powerful ways to maintain not only physical strength but also mental clarity and emotional resilience. Staying active helps keep the body strong and mobile, your mind sharp, and your spirit light. This isn't about achieving perfection or pushing limits; it's about taking steps to improve your quality of life and investing in a future filled with vitality and independence. Every walk around the neighborhood, every stretch before bed, and every strengthening exercise is a step toward freedom—freedom to move with ease, handle everyday tasks, and engage in the activities you love.

You may wonder where to start or what to focus on first, and that's why this book is structured to meet you where you are. With carefully chosen exercises that address strength, balance, flexibility, and cardiovascular health, each chapter guides you through movements designed to support you in living fully, on your own terms. In the following pages, you'll find exercises that cater to all levels, with simple instructions that make every movement feel accessible and manageable. This book is more than an exercise guide—it's a resource to help you build confidence, encouraging you to move forward with each chapter.

In the back of the book, you'll find an appendix that serves as a handy reference for the exercises mentioned. Here, you'll see all the exercises listed alphabetically, complete with detailed instructions, tips for proper form, and variations to suit your needs. This section includes helpful illustrations to guide you visually, so you can feel confident in performing each movement safely and effectively. The appendix is there to support you whenever you need a quick reminder, whether you're practicing balance, building strength, or simply exploring new ways to keep active.

Remember, this journey isn't about comparing yourself to others or aiming for unreachable milestones. It's about celebrating what your body can achieve, honoring the resilience it has shown, and nurturing it with kindness. Embrace each small success as a victory, knowing that with every movement, you're investing in a healthier, more vibrant life. So take a deep breath, turn the page, and let's embark on this journey together. Here's to stronger days, lighter steps, and a life lived to the fullest.

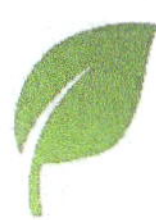

Understanding the Importance of Exercise After 60

The advantages of regular physical activity extend far beyond the obvious physical health benefits. For seniors, staying active is crucial in maintaining mental acuity, emotional well-being, and overall quality of life. Engaging in regular exercise helps to manage and prevent age-related diseases such as heart disease, diabetes, and osteoporosis. It also significantly boosts mental health, helping to ward off age-related cognitive decline and symptoms of depression and anxiety.

Physical activity increases stamina and strength, enabling you to continue performing everyday tasks independently. Whether it's gardening, walking the dog, or playing with grandchildren, exercise ensures that you can continue these activities with ease and less fatigue. Moreover, social interactions during group exercises or community walks can lead to lasting friendships, enhancing social networks that are often at risk as one ages.

Common Health Concerns Addressed Through Exercise

Regular exercise is one of the most effective ways to address and mitigate common health concerns that arise with age. For instance, weight-bearing exercises such as walking or gentle weight training can improve bone density and help combat osteoporosis. Strength training enhances muscle mass, which naturally declines with age, reducing the risk of falls and improving overall mobility.

Cardiovascular exercises like swimming or cycling are vital in managing hypertension and reducing the risk of heart disease. Additionally, flexibility and balance exercises such as yoga or Tai Chi can prevent falls—a major concern for aging adults—by improving coordination and balance.

Exercise also plays a crucial role in pain management, particularly for conditions like arthritis. Regular movement keeps joints fluid and can help reduce overall pain levels associated with inflammatory conditions.

Committing to Your Health

As you embark on this fitness journey, remember that it is never too late to start. The exercises included in this book have been carefully selected and adapted to suit a wide range of physical capabilities and health considerations typical of seniors over 60. Each activity is designed to be safe, enjoyable, and beneficial, regardless of your current fitness level.

In the comprehensive appendix of this book, you will find detailed descriptions of all the exercises mentioned throughout the chapters. They are presented in alphabetical order to ease navigation and include variants and tips to tailor each activity to your needs. This section ensures that you have all the information at your fingertips, helping you to perform each exercise correctly and safely. Detailed illustrations accompany these descriptions, providing visual cues that enhance understanding and execution.

This guide is more than just an exercise manual; it's a blueprint for a more vibrant and active lifestyle in your

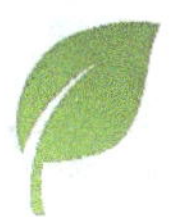

senior years. It empowers you to take charge of your health, offering tools and knowledge that enable you to make informed decisions about your physical activity.

The design of this book considers ease of reading, avoiding overly complex terminology or dense sections that could detract from the learning experience. Our goal is to make the information as accessible and actionable as possible, allowing you to integrate these exercises into your daily routine seamlessly.

As you progress, you may find yourself capable of more than you thought possible, opening doors to new activities and perhaps even new friendships. Exercise is a celebration of what your body can do, and this book is here to guide you every step of the way.

Embark on this journey with confidence, knowing that each step you take is a step towards a healthier, more fulfilling life. Here's to your health, strength, and happiness—let's get moving!

This introduction is designed to be informative and motivational, addressing the physical, mental, and social aspects of exercising in later life while ensuring it is approachable and directly applicable to the reader's daily life.

Physical benefits of exercising in your 60s

For women in their 60s, staying active can feel like reclaiming a bit of freedom. Exercise isn't just about working up a sweat—it's a powerful way to keep your heart strong, your body steady, and your bones resilient, so you can stay engaged in the activities you love and enjoy each day with

confidence. Let's dive into how even simple movements can work wonders on your body.

Heart health is so important as we age. Did you know that even a brisk walk around the neighborhood or a bit of gardening can be like a gift to your heart? Regular, gentle exercises help lower blood pressure and manage cholesterol, keeping your heart strong and lowering your risk of heart disease. Think of these moments as a way to nurture the very part of you that keeps everything going. Many women your age have shared how daily walks or a few minutes on a stationary bike have given them renewed energy—and more peace of mind.

Aging naturally brings changes to our muscles, but it doesn't mean we have to sit back and accept the loss of strength. Simple strength-building exercises, like lifting light weights or using resistance bands, can help keep your muscles active and engaged. This means you'll be able to carry your groceries, play with your grandkids, or even tackle those household chores with more ease. Mary, 64, from Ohio, shared that adding a few squats and leg lifts to her morning routine helped her feel "stronger and capable" in a way she hadn't felt in years. Small steps lead to big rewards, and just a few minutes each day can keep your muscles ready to support you.

For many women, the fear of falls and fractures is all too real. Bones naturally become more fragile as we age, but you can strengthen yours with weight-bearing exercises. Walking, low-impact aerobics, or gentle dance moves encourage your bones to stay strong and support you. Think of these movements as part of a toolkit that helps you continue doing what you love with confidence. Imagine yourself feeling more balanced and steady, reducing that

fear of falls. Women like Janet, who took up dancing classes, found that her posture and balance improved within a few months—plus, she had fun along the way!

Keeping an active metabolism becomes more challenging in our 60s, but physical activity can be a game-changer. Exercise helps manage blood sugar levels, reduce inflammation, and keep weight in check. These benefits protect you from common age-related issues, like diabetes, that can disrupt daily life. Many seniors find that by mixing a little strength work with gentle cardio, they feel more in control of their health and energy levels. It's not about keeping up with anyone else—just creating a routine that feels right for you.

At the heart of it all, staying active means staying independent. Being able to move freely, handle your own errands, and enjoy your favorite hobbies without help is a priceless gift to yourself. Imagine yourself feeling steady and secure with each step, free from the worries of needing extra help. Think of these exercises as tools to keep you connected to the life you enjoy, with the people you care about, and to the moments that bring you joy.

So remember, this isn't about achieving perfection—it's about taking small steps toward a life that feels strong, steady, and fulfilling. Embrace each step as an act of caring for yourself and celebrating what your body can still do. You're not just staying active; you're giving yourself the freedom to continue living life on your terms.

Mental and Emotional Benefits of Staying Active

Staying active isn't just about keeping our bodies strong—it's about nurturing our minds and spirits, too. For women

in their 60s, exercise can be a powerful way to boost mood, calm anxieties, and even support memory and focus. Imagine each movement as a gift to yourself, helping you find more peace and joy in everyday life.

Exercise has a unique ability to lift our spirits. When we move our bodies, even in gentle ways like stretching or walking, our brains release "feel-good" chemicals that naturally improve mood. Some women say that a short walk outdoors, breathing in fresh air and feeling the sun on their face, is enough to turn a difficult day around. Activities like yoga or tai chi can help you feel grounded and centered, turning exercise into a time of peace and positivity. For women like Linda, who began a daily stretching routine at 62, these small movements felt like a way to nurture her mind as much as her body, helping her start each day with calm and gratitude.

Reducing Stress and Anxiety

Life in our 60s comes with its own set of worries—about health, family, finances, and sometimes even loneliness. Exercise is a wonderful way to handle these feelings. Gentle movement, whether it's a few stretches, a bike ride, or even chair yoga, helps us release built-up tension. Studies show that physical activity lowers levels of stress hormones and brings a sense of calm. Many women find that a few mindful movements each day help them feel more at ease and in control. Take Joyce, for instance; she found that a few minutes of yoga each morning helped her keep stress at bay and face her day with a clearer mind.

Staying active can also help keep our minds sharp. Research shows that exercise supports healthy blood flow to the brain, which is key for memory and cognitive

function. Activities that require coordination, like balance exercises or even learning a new dance move, challenge the brain and keep it engaged. Think of these activities as exercise for the mind as well as the body. Simple routines that include coordination—like walking heel-to-toe or balancing on one leg—can have surprising benefits for mental focus. Carol, 64, shared how practicing balance moves not only helped her stability but made her feel "more alert and mentally agile" in her day-to-day activities.

Exercise also plays a big role in improving sleep. Good sleep is vital for energy and mood, yet many women find restful nights hard to come by. Regular physical activity can help regulate sleep patterns, making it easier to fall asleep and stay asleep. Even gentle exercises, like an evening walk or a simple stretching routine, help the body wind down for a good night's rest. Sarah, who struggled with sleep issues for years, discovered that a relaxing stretch routine before bed helped her feel calm and ready for sleep.

There's something deeply satisfying about moving our bodies, even in the simplest ways. Each time you finish a routine or try a new movement, it's a reminder of your strength and resilience. Exercise can be a celebration of what our bodies can still do and a way to connect to a sense of joy and achievement. With each step, each stretch, and each breath, you're taking care of your mind and spirit, keeping them as healthy and strong as your body.

So, as you begin this journey, remember that each movement brings more than physical benefits—it's a gift to your mental and emotional health, helping you feel more positive, more centered, and more connected to the life you love.

Quality of Life: Living Fully and Independently

Embracing Movement to Enhance Everyday Moments

For many women in their 60s, staying active is about more than just fitness—it's about protecting and enhancing the quality of life we've built over the years. Exercise helps us keep doing the things that bring joy, allow us to connect with others, and let us move confidently through the world.

Physical activity can be a bridge to meaningful moments. Imagine feeling steady enough to keep up with grandkids, take a stroll with friends, or work in the garden without feeling held back. A simple, regular movement routine can keep these experiences accessible. Many women share that by committing to even a few minutes of activity, they can keep engaging in these everyday moments.

Exercise also strengthens our connections. From walking with a friend to joining a local exercise group, movement brings us closer to those around us. Mary, for instance, started taking morning walks with her neighbor, and the combination of gentle activity and companionship brought new joy and connection to her days.

There's also the priceless satisfaction of maintaining independence. When we can rely on our bodies, we're free to live life on our own terms. Carrying groceries, navigating stairs, or reaching for items on a high shelf— exercise gives us the strength to manage these daily activities independently. This self-sufficiency is more than physical; it's deeply empowering.

On top of that, exercise can ease stress and add calm to our routines. Movement helps us stay present, releasing

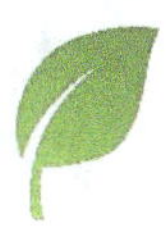

the worries that can sometimes cloud our thoughts. Life brings challenges and changes, but exercise offers a steadying force that lets us feel grounded.

So as you begin your exercise journey, remember that each movement is an investment in your quality of life. These efforts will ripple through your connections, your independence, and your sense of joy. Embrace this opportunity to live fully, with all the richness and resilience it brings. You're giving yourself the gift of freedom, strength, and fulfillment in every moment.

Common Health Concerns Addressed Through Exercise

Supporting Your Body's Needs

As we enter our 60s, certain health concerns become more prevalent, and exercise can be one of the best ways to address them. For women in this age group, physical activity isn't about pushing limits but about supporting and listening to the body. Whether it's managing arthritis, keeping the heart strong, or preventing falls, staying active helps us age with strength and confidence.

Arthritis is a common concern for many women, often bringing joint stiffness and discomfort. Fortunately, gentle, low-impact movements can be a real remedy. Exercises like walking, swimming, and even simple seated stretching routines reduce joint pain by increasing blood flow to the area, which helps keep joints flexible and reduces inflammation. Many women have found that just a few minutes of movement each day makes a noticeable difference. Anne, a 65-year-old with arthritis in her knees, shared that after starting a gentle stretching and

resistance routine, her knees felt less stiff, and she found herself moving more freely and confidently around the house.

Heart health also takes center stage as we age. Post-menopause, women have an increased risk of heart disease, so staying active is key. Cardiovascular exercises, such as brisk walking or light cycling, work wonders for heart health, and they don't need to be high-intensity to be effective. Regular movement helps to lower blood pressure, improve cholesterol levels, and boost energy, contributing to a healthier heart. Mary, a vibrant 63-year-old, found that her daily morning walks helped her feel energized and offered peace of mind, knowing she was doing something valuable for her heart every day.

Balance and fall prevention are particularly important for women in their 60s, as fall-related injuries can impact independence. Exercises that improve balance, such as standing on one leg or practicing heel-to-toe walking, strengthen the stabilizing muscles and give you a greater sense of control and coordination. Just a few minutes of balance work each day can make a real difference in feeling steady. Linda, who'd become cautious about her footing, found that these balance exercises gave her a new sense of confidence, whether walking up the stairs or reaching for something high on a shelf.

Flexibility and mobility exercises—such as gentle stretching, yoga, or Pilates—help maintain a wide range of motion, making everyday movements easier and more comfortable. The more flexible we are, the more easily we can bend, reach, and navigate daily activities. Think of these exercises as small, preventive steps that keep the body feeling free and agile. For many women, these

movements are a game-changer; they reduce stiffness and make tasks like tying shoes or reaching up into a cabinet feel easier.

Exercise is a tool for supporting health and addressing the unique needs that come with age. Embracing a routine, even a simple one, brings physical relief and a sense of empowerment and resilience. So, whether you're starting with short walks, a gentle stretch, or a few minutes of balance work, remember that each movement is an investment in your well-being, helping your body support you as you live fully and independently. Every step, stretch, and mindful movement matters—each one bringing you closer to feeling strong, capable, and at ease in your own body.

Setting Expectations

Building a Routine, One Step at a Time

Starting or returning to an exercise routine after 60 can be both exciting and a little intimidating. The journey to better health and mobility doesn't happen overnight, and it's important to set realistic, achievable goals that honor where you are right now. This chapter is all about setting those expectations so you feel motivated and empowered, not overwhelmed.

Many women come to exercise with the hope of feeling stronger, more energized, or simply more capable in their daily lives. These are wonderful goals, and with a bit of patience and consistency, they are absolutely attainable. But it's also helpful to remember that progress may look different now than it did in our younger years—and that's

okay. This is a time to listen to your body and move at your own pace, celebrating each small victory along the way.

One of the first steps in building a lasting routine is to start small. Begin with exercises that feel comfortable and manageable. This could be as simple as a 5-minute walk, a few gentle stretches, or even balance exercises that you can do right from your living room. The goal isn't to push yourself to exhaustion but to create a routine that you can look forward to. Each small step builds on the last, creating a foundation of strength, flexibility, and confidence that will serve you over time.

It's also helpful to set goals that focus on consistency rather than intensity. For instance, aim to incorporate some form of movement into your daily life—whether it's a short walk, a gentle yoga session, or even household activities like gardening or tidying up. As you create a rhythm of daily movement, you'll notice that your body responds positively, and activities that once seemed challenging may feel easier over time.

There may be days when movement feels more difficult, and that's natural. Life has its ups and downs, and so will your fitness journey. When this happens, give yourself grace. Even a small amount of movement—such as a light stretch or a short stroll—can make a difference. The key is to keep moving, even if it's in a gentler way than usual.

Another important aspect of setting expectations is to focus on your personal journey rather than comparing yourself to others. Everyone's body and experience are different. What matters is finding what works best for you, so you can feel confident and supported in your routine. Remember, every woman in this book, and every expert

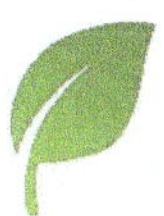

who shares advice, started somewhere. They, too, have had days of doubt and challenges to overcome.

As you begin your journey, keep these expectations in mind. Each step, no matter how small, is a victory worth celebrating. You're building a foundation for a healthier, more independent future, and every effort you make brings you closer to that goal. Embrace each day as it comes, honoring your progress and remembering that the journey to wellness is about progress, not perfection. You've got this—one step at a time.

Conclusion of the Introduction

As you embark on this journey to a healthier, more active life, remember that every step you take—no matter how small—is an investment in yourself. This book is here to guide you, encourage you, and remind you that you're capable of so much. Embracing movement at this stage of life is an act of self-care, resilience, and empowerment. It's a way to honor your body, nurture your spirit, and create a future filled with independence, joy, and vitality.

You may face challenges along the way, but know that they're simply part of the journey. Each chapter of this book is crafted to support you in building a routine that fits your lifestyle, meets you where you are, and grows with you over time. From practical advice to inspiring stories and expert insights, this guide is filled with tools to help you thrive.

So take a deep breath, set aside any worries, and focus on what you can do today. Whether it's a gentle stretch, a walk around the block, or simply reading these words, you're already taking positive steps forward. This journey

is yours to enjoy, and every bit of effort brings you closer to a healthier, more vibrant life. Let's begin, with gratitude for where we are and excitement for what's to come.

CHAPTER 1:

PREPARING FOR EXERCISE

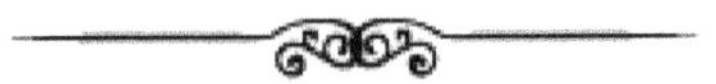

1.1 Consultation with Health Professionals

Starting a new exercise routine in your 60s is a powerful step toward enhancing your strength, independence, and overall well-being. But before diving into a new program, it's important to connect with your healthcare providers. This initial step is like setting up a strong foundation for your journey, ensuring you're well-informed and equipped to exercise safely and effectively.

Health professionals, such as doctors and physical therapists, are valuable allies in this process. They can offer insights into any health conditions that might influence your routine, such as arthritis, high blood pressure, or osteoporosis. These conditions don't necessarily limit your ability to exercise but can shape how you approach certain activities. For example, if you have arthritis, your doctor may suggest low-impact activities like walking, swimming, or chair exercises, which protect your joints while still providing the benefits of movement.

Meeting with a doctor or physical therapist also allows you to discuss any questions or concerns you might have. If you're uncertain about the intensity level that's safe for

you, they can provide guidance on where to start and how to gradually increase your activity over time. Likewise, if you have concerns about monitoring your heart rate, balance, or endurance, healthcare professionals can guide you in using methods and tools that enhance safety and confidence.

Physical therapists, in particular, can be invaluable for designing a personalized exercise plan that caters to your specific needs. They can identify muscle imbalances, areas of weakness, or joint concerns that may benefit from specific strengthening or flexibility exercises. Their expertise helps create a plan that aligns with your goals while respecting your body's current capabilities.

Taking the time to consult with a healthcare provider before starting an exercise routine brings peace of mind. Knowing that your plan is tailored to support your body, rather than work against it, allows you to begin with confidence and positivity. This proactive approach is all about setting yourself up for long-term success, empowering you to embrace a healthier, more active lifestyle with the reassurance that your routine is safe, effective, and supportive of your individual needs.

As you move forward, remember that this foundation is your anchor. Consulting with healthcare providers isn't just a one-time event; it's an ongoing resource. Over time, as your fitness levels and goals evolve, consider checking back in with your providers to ensure your exercise plan continues to align with your needs.

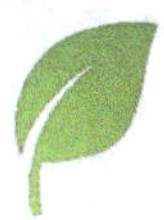

1.2 Setting Up Your Exercise Space

Creating an exercise space that's comfortable, safe, and inviting can be a huge motivator for staying active. This doesn't mean you need a full home gym; a simple setup can be just as effective. The goal is to make sure you have a designated area where you feel ready to move, free from distractions or hazards, and equipped with the basics you need to exercise confidently.

Choosing the Right Spot

Start by selecting a spot in your home that has enough space for you to move comfortably. This could be a corner in your living room, a section of your bedroom, or even a quiet area in the basement. Aim for a spot where you can stretch out without bumping into furniture, and ensure it's free of any potential tripping hazards, like loose rugs or cords. Good lighting is also key, especially if you're following an exercise guide or video, as it helps you stay clear and focused on your movements.

Gathering Your Equipment

You don't need a lot of fancy equipment, but a few basic items can make your workout experience smoother and more enjoyable. Light hand weights, resistance bands, and a sturdy chair for balance exercises are all simple additions that can enhance your routine. If you prefer body-weight exercises or stretching, a comfortable yoga mat can be a great asset, offering support and preventing slipping on hard floors. And if balance is a concern, having a nearby wall or counter for extra support can give you that extra bit of stability when you need it.

A welcoming space goes a long way in making exercise feel like a positive part of your day. Small touches like a favorite playlist, natural lighting, or even a houseplant can help create an environment that feels inviting and uplifting. Some people enjoy diffusing calming essential oils, like lavender or eucalyptus, to make their space feel relaxing and fresh. You could also keep a water bottle, towel, or small fan nearby to stay comfortable throughout your session.

Safety is a top priority when setting up your exercise space. Make sure your area is clear of anything that could cause a trip or slip. For floor exercises, choose a mat that won't slide, and if you're using weights, keep them on a stable surface. It's also a good idea to have a phone or emergency alert device nearby, especially if you're exercising alone. These small precautions allow you to move confidently, knowing you're prepared and protected.

Setting Yourself Up for Success

Finally, think about how to make your space feel like your own. This is your area for growth, strength, and health, so personalize it in a way that brings you joy. Some people like to keep an exercise journal nearby to track their progress, while others enjoy adding inspiring quotes or photos that remind them of their goals. Creating a space that feels special to you can make it easier to return each day, transforming exercise into a habit that you look forward to.

Setting up a dedicated exercise space doesn't have to be complicated. With a few thoughtful touches, you'll have a comfortable, practical spot where you can focus on your fitness journey. This small investment in your

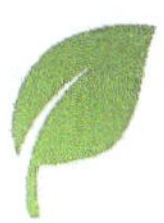

surroundings can make a big difference in your motivation, helping you approach each session with positivity and enthusiasm.

1.3 Essential Equipment for Home Workouts

Exercising at home is both convenient and comfortable, and with just a few pieces of equipment, you can create a well-rounded workout routine right where you are. The goal isn't to have an entire gym setup but rather a few versatile tools that can help you build strength, improve flexibility, and enhance balance. Here's a look at some essential, senior-friendly equipment to support your fitness journey.

Light Hand Weights

Hand weights, often referred to as dumbbells, are incredibly versatile and effective for building muscle strength. When starting out, look for light weights, usually around 1 to 5 pounds, that allow you to complete exercises comfortably. Hand weights are great for exercises like bicep curls, shoulder presses, and even some balance exercises. They help you build upper body strength, which is essential for everyday tasks like lifting, reaching, and carrying. Remember, you can always increase weight as you feel stronger and more confident.

Resistance Bands

Resistance bands are an excellent tool for gentle, low-impact strength training. These stretchy bands come in various levels of resistance, so you can choose the one that feels best for you. They're gentle on the joints and can be used for exercises targeting every part of the body,

from arms and shoulders to legs and glutes. What's great about resistance bands is their flexibility; they're light, portable, and easy to use even in small spaces. Plus, they're effective for both beginners and more advanced fitness levels.

Chair or Sturdy Support

For balance exercises and seated workouts, a sturdy chair or support like a countertop can be incredibly helpful. A chair provides a stable base for exercises that improve balance, flexibility, and lower body strength. For example, it's ideal for seated leg lifts, stretching, or using for balance in standing exercises. When choosing a chair, make sure it's stable, without wheels, and the right height for you. Having a sturdy support nearby can also boost confidence, giving you something to hold onto when practicing balance moves.

Yoga or Exercise Mat

A comfortable, non-slip mat is a wonderful addition to your exercise space, especially for floor exercises and stretches. Mats provide cushioning for your joints, making movements like stretching, seated exercises, or even gentle yoga more comfortable on hard floors. Look for a mat with good grip, especially if you're working on balance exercises. A quality mat adds stability and makes each exercise feel more grounded.

Other Useful Additions

While not essential, other items like a foam roller, exercise ball, or ankle weights can enhance certain exercises and provide variety. Foam rollers are fantastic for relieving

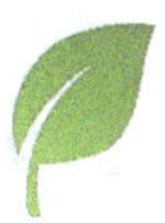

muscle tension and promoting flexibility, especially if you're easing into a new routine. An exercise ball can be used for seated exercises and gentle stretching, while ankle weights add a bit more challenge to leg exercises.

With just a few simple items, you'll have all you need to stay strong, flexible, and balanced. Remember, equipment doesn't have to be fancy or extensive—just functional. Choose pieces that feel comfortable and accessible, and add new items over time as you feel ready. This way, your home becomes a supportive space for movement, giving you everything you need to enjoy a safe, effective workout routine tailored just for you.

1.4 Understanding Your Body's Limits

Starting an exercise routine in your 60s is about finding a balance that allows you to embrace movement while respecting your body's unique needs. Knowing your limits isn't a barrier; it's a way to create a routine that brings real benefits without overexertion. Exercise can be deeply rewarding when done with mindfulness and care.

The first step is learning to listen to your body. Each time you exercise, take a moment to notice how you feel. Some days, you may be full of energy, while on others, you might need to take things a little slower. By tuning into these signals, you can adjust your intensity as needed, making each workout feel comfortable and beneficial. Pain or discomfort during an exercise is a sign to pause or modify—exercise should feel positive, not forced or painful.

Starting slowly and building gradually is also key to long-term success. While it's exciting to begin a new routine,

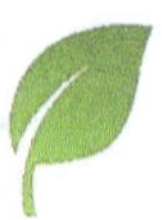

pacing yourself is essential. Begin with shorter sessions and simpler exercises to give your muscles and joints time to adapt. Over time, you'll build strength and endurance, making it easier to increase your activity level without strain.

Modifying and Celebrating Progress

Modifications can help create a routine that fits you. If a standing exercise feels challenging, try a seated version. If lifting weights feels too intense, begin with body-weight exercises until you feel ready for more. Tailoring each exercise to meet your needs allows you to participate fully and comfortably. Many women find that adapting exercises lets them experience the benefits without overdoing it.

Rest and recovery are essential to a well-rounded routine. Exercise challenges your muscles and joints, and resting allows them to heal and strengthen. On days when you feel sore or tired, consider taking a rest day or focusing on gentle stretching. Rest days prevent burnout and help keep you energized for the journey ahead.

Finally, remember to celebrate each small victory. Whether it's finishing a workout, feeling more energetic, or simply showing up for yourself, each step is progress. By respecting your limits, you're building a routine that's safe and empowering, helping you enjoy this journey without feeling rushed or pressured.

Understanding your limits allows you to exercise with confidence and joy, supporting your health in a way that feels right for you. This mindful approach makes exercise a positive experience, helping you stay active and engaged while caring for yourself in the best way possible.

CHAPTER 2

SAFETY FIRST

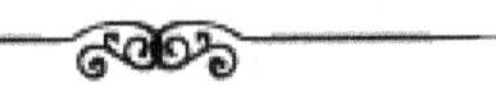

2.1 Warming Up Properly

Warming up is an essential part of any exercise routine, especially as we get older. A good warm-up gently prepares your body for movement, loosening up muscles and increasing circulation. This is your body's signal that it's time to get moving, helping you ease into exercise with comfort and confidence. Think of it as setting the stage for a safe, effective workout.

Warming up doesn't need to be intense or lengthy. In fact, just 5 to 10 minutes of gentle movement can make a noticeable difference in how your body feels. Start with simple activities that gradually raise your heart rate, like gentle marching in place or slow arm circles. This kind of low-intensity movement warms up your muscles, increases blood flow, and starts lubricating your joints, which can help prevent stiffness and reduce the risk of injury.

Stretching as part of your warm-up can also be beneficial, especially for muscles that may feel tight, like those in the shoulders, lower back, and legs. Dynamic stretches, which involve gentle, controlled movements, are ideal for warming up. For example, slow leg swings, torso twists, or gentle

shoulder rolls are excellent choices. These stretches aren't about pushing your limits but rather about loosening up, so you feel prepared for the activity ahead.

Moving at Your Own Pace

Remember, warming up is your time to ease into movement, so listen to your body and take it at your own pace. If something feels uncomfortable, don't push it—simply shift to a movement that feels good. The goal is to bring warmth and flexibility to your muscles, setting you up for a positive exercise experience. A good warm-up helps you enter each workout with more ease, ensuring that you feel ready, relaxed, and focused on the steps ahead.

For many women, the warm-up becomes a cherished part of the routine, a few moments to connect with their bodies and tune in to how they're feeling. It's also a reminder that exercise doesn't have to start with intensity; sometimes, the most gentle movements can be the most impactful in setting a strong foundation.

So as you prepare for each workout, embrace the warm-up as a valuable part of the process. You're giving your body the care it deserves, making sure that every step, stretch, and lift that follows feels comfortable and supported. Warming up may be a small part of your routine, but it's one of the most important steps you can take toward a safe, enjoyable, and rewarding fitness journey.

2.2 Preventing Injuries

Preventing injuries is one of the most important aspects of building a safe and sustainable exercise routine. When we're young, our bodies may recover more easily from

occasional strain, but as we age, it's essential to be proactive about protecting our muscles, joints, and bones. Injury prevention isn't just about avoiding setbacks—it's about building confidence and maintaining consistency in your fitness journey.

One of the best ways to prevent injuries is by paying attention to your form. Proper form ensures that you're using your body efficiently and reduces unnecessary stress on your muscles and joints. Start each movement with intention, focusing on alignment and control. For example, when doing a squat, keep your feet firmly planted, engage your core, and avoid letting your knees move inward. If you're unsure of the correct form, consider starting with exercises that use a mirror, or even ask for guidance from a professional if you're able. Practicing proper form may take time, but it will serve you well in the long run.

Listening to your body is another crucial part of injury prevention. Some exercises might feel challenging, but they should never cause pain. If you feel any sharp or intense discomfort, stop immediately and reassess. Adjust the movement, switch to a gentler exercise, or take a rest. It's natural for our bodies to have occasional limitations, and there's no need to push through discomfort. Knowing when to pause is an act of self-care and respect for your body's boundaries.

Injury prevention also involves allowing your body time to rest and recover. Even when you're eager to stay active, rest days are essential for muscle repair and growth. Over time, this balance between activity and recovery helps you build resilience, keeping your body strong and ready for each session. On rest days, gentle activities like

stretching, walking, or yoga can still be beneficial, as they promote circulation and relaxation without overloading your muscles.

Adding variety to your routine can also help protect you from overuse injuries, which occur when the same muscles are repeatedly stressed. Incorporate a mix of activities like strength training, stretching, balance work, and light cardio to give different parts of your body the chance to rest and recharge. Variety keeps your muscles engaged and challenged, while reducing the risk of repetitive strain.

Injury prevention isn't about avoiding challenges—it's about making thoughtful choices that support your health and keep you moving forward. By focusing on form, listening to your body, incorporating rest, and varying your routine, you're creating a foundation that not only keeps you safe but also helps you grow stronger over time. Embrace these steps as part of your journey, knowing that each one supports a more fulfilling and empowering approach to fitness.

2.3 When to Stop – Recognizing Your Body's Signals

Listening to your body and recognizing when to stop is a vital skill for maintaining a long-term, injury-free exercise routine. As we age, our bodies may require more time to recover, and it's important to acknowledge when rest is needed. While pushing ourselves to achieve goals is important, it's just as essential to respect our limits and recognize when we've done enough for the day. This doesn't mean you're not strong or capable—it's about giving your body the care and attention it deserves so that

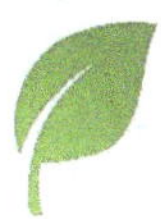

you can continue moving safely and effectively in the long run.

During exercise, your body will naturally send you signals that indicate when to stop or slow down. These signals can include feelings of dizziness, shortness of breath, sharp pain, or even extreme fatigue. These signs should never be ignored. If you feel any of these, it's important to stop immediately, rest, and reassess how you're feeling. Even if it's just a slight discomfort, take it as a cue to pause. Pushing through pain or discomfort can lead to longer recovery times or injury, which can derail your progress entirely. Instead, stop, breathe deeply, and listen to what your body is trying to tell you.

It's also important to distinguish between the normal discomfort that comes from exerting effort and the pain that signals a potential injury. Discomfort during exercise, such as feeling slightly winded or sore in the muscles, is completely normal, especially if you're challenging yourself. This kind of discomfort is usually temporary and will subside after rest. However, pain is a different story. Pain, especially sharp or intense, can be a warning sign of a strain or injury. If you experience pain in your joints, muscles, or bones, stop the exercise immediately and consider modifying your routine.

Another sign to look for is if your body begins to feel off balance or uncoordinated. Dizziness or lightheadedness can indicate that you're overexerting yourself. If you notice these symptoms, sit down, drink some water, and take a few deep breaths. If the feelings persist, it's a good idea to seek advice from a health professional to ensure your fitness plan is right for your current health status.

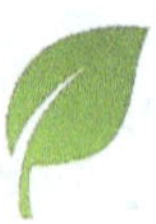

Taking Breaks and Hydration

During your exercise session, be sure to take breaks as needed. If you're doing a cardio workout, it's especially important to listen for signs of fatigue or breathlessness. Taking regular, short breaks helps your body maintain its energy levels and can prevent overexertion. If you feel your energy dipping, don't hesitate to slow down or rest for a moment. Hydration is equally important, as dehydration can contribute to feelings of dizziness or discomfort. Always have water nearby and take sips throughout your routine to stay hydrated.

It's equally important to recognize the importance of rest days in your fitness routine. While daily exercise can be great, rest is a crucial part of the process. Giving your muscles and joints time to recover ensures you don't overtax your body and helps to avoid burnout. Many people underestimate how important recovery is, but without it, progress can be limited. Aim to take at least one or two rest days a week to give your body the time it needs to repair itself.

Recognizing when to stop and when to modify your routine is about self-care and listening to the wisdom of your body. By paying attention to your body's signals, you can prevent injury, improve your fitness journey, and enjoy the long-term benefits of staying active. Respecting your limits doesn't mean stopping progress—it means moving forward in a way that's sustainable and healthy for you.

2.4 Cooling Down and Recovery

After a workout, cooling down is just as important as warming up. It's your body's way of gradually transitioning

from physical activity to a state of rest, helping to prevent injury and reduce muscle soreness. Cooling down also promotes relaxation, allowing your heart rate to return to normal and helping your body recover more effectively after exercise. Just like warming up, cooling down doesn't need to be long or complicated—just a few gentle movements can make a big difference.

Start by reducing the intensity of your workout slowly. For instance, if you've been walking or doing light cardio, slow your pace for the last few minutes. This gradual reduction helps your heart rate decrease safely, preventing dizziness or lightheadedness that can occur if you stop suddenly. If you've been doing strength exercises, follow them with some light stretching to bring flexibility back into your muscles. Gently stretching your arms, legs, and back will help release any tightness that's built up during the session.

Cooling down is also an excellent time to practice deep breathing. Breathing deeply helps reduce stress, calm the mind, and improve oxygen flow throughout the body. Take slow, deep breaths, inhaling through your nose and exhaling through your mouth. This not only helps lower your heart rate but also promotes a sense of calm, leaving you feeling refreshed and at ease after the workout.

Listening to Your Body During Recovery

Just as it's important to listen to your body during the workout, it's crucial to continue doing so during your recovery period. After a workout, you may feel tired, and that's completely normal. However, if you experience pain or persistent discomfort, it may be a sign that you've overdone it. If you feel any sharp pain during the cooldown

or afterwards, take extra time to rest and recover. On those days, avoid intense physical activity and focus on gentle stretching or even just walking.

Recovery isn't just about cooling down after exercise; it's an ongoing process that includes getting enough sleep, staying hydrated, and allowing your muscles time to repair. Rest is essential, especially as we age, and giving your body the time it needs to recover will ensure that you're ready to tackle your next workout with energy and enthusiasm.

Hydration and Nutrition

Another important aspect of recovery is staying hydrated. Drinking water after exercise helps replace the fluids lost through sweat and supports muscle recovery. If your workout was particularly intense or lasted for a long period, consider sipping on an electrolyte-rich drink to replenish lost minerals. Nutrition also plays a key role in recovery. Eating a balanced meal or snack with protein and healthy carbs within an hour of exercising can help repair muscles and restore your energy levels.

Taking these simple but effective steps—cooling down, staying hydrated, and eating well—can make a significant difference in how you feel the next day. With consistent recovery practices, you'll notice improvements in flexibility, energy, and overall strength. Incorporating this time for your body to rest and heal is just as important as the workout itself and sets the foundation for continued progress.

Cooling down and recovery are opportunities to honor the hard work your body has done. By making recovery a

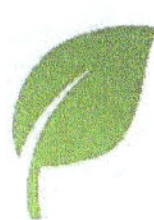

priority, you're ensuring that you're not only avoiding injury but also enhancing your ability to stay active and engaged in the long term. It's all part of taking care of yourself, building strength, and maintaining a healthy, sustainable fitness routine that fits your lifestyle.

CHAPTER 3

EXERCISES FOR EVERYONE

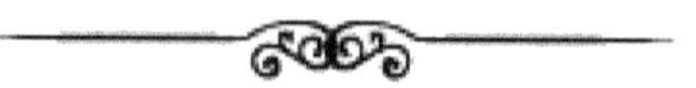

3.1 Gentle Stretching Routines to Enhance Flexibility

Flexibility is one of the most important aspects of maintaining mobility and preventing injury as we age. A good stretching routine not only improves flexibility but also promotes circulation, reduces muscle stiffness, and can even enhance your mood. For women in their 60s, gentle stretching is an excellent way to stay mobile and enjoy a greater range of motion in everyday activities, from bending down to tie your shoes to reaching for something on a high shelf.

Stretching can be incorporated into your daily routine, and it doesn't need to be time-consuming or strenuous. A few minutes each day is enough to experience the benefits. The key is consistency, rather than intensity. The goal of stretching isn't to push your body to its limits but to gently ease into the movement and listen to what feels right. Stretching should never cause pain, but it can help release tight muscles and improve your posture and mobility over time.

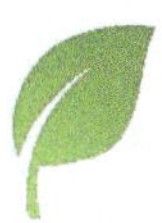

Start with simple, low-impact stretches that target areas where tension tends to build up, like the lower back, hips, shoulders, and legs. You can perform these stretches while seated or standing, depending on what feels most comfortable for you. For example, seated hamstring stretches, gentle side stretches, and shoulder rolls are all effective ways to ease tension without putting undue stress on your body.

It's important to remember that stretching is a slow and controlled process. Hold each stretch for 15 to 30 seconds and take slow, deep breaths to help your muscles relax. If you feel any discomfort, ease off the stretch and never force your body into a deeper position. Over time, as your flexibility improves, you may find that you can increase the duration of each stretch or go a bit deeper, but this should be done gradually.

Targeting Key Areas

The most common areas that benefit from gentle stretching are the back, legs, hips, and shoulders. For example, a seated spinal twist can help open up the spine and improve posture, while a calf stretch can help with ankle flexibility and mobility. A gentle stretch for the hip flexors can alleviate tightness from sitting for long periods, which is common as we age. By regularly stretching these areas, you can improve your overall flexibility, making everyday movements feel easier and more comfortable.

Incorporating flexibility exercises into your routine is a simple yet effective way to enhance your mobility and prevent stiffness. As you develop a consistent stretching practice, you'll find that you feel more energized and physically capable. Stretching is a gentle way to keep your

body moving fluidly, helping you maintain independence and enjoy all the activities you love. So take the time to stretch daily—your body will thank you.

3.2 Cardiovascular Exercises for Heart Health

Cardiovascular exercise, often referred to as cardio, is essential for maintaining a healthy heart, and it offers a wide range of benefits for seniors. As we age, our cardiovascular system naturally weakens, but regular aerobic exercise helps counteract this decline. For women in their 60s, engaging in heart-healthy activities not only reduces the risk of heart disease and stroke but also improves stamina, lung capacity, and overall energy levels, making it easier to engage in daily activities.

The great thing about cardio is that it doesn't have to mean running marathons or intense gym workouts. Cardiovascular exercises can be simple, low-impact activities that fit easily into your daily routine. Walking, swimming, cycling, or even dancing are all excellent options for getting your heart rate up while being gentle on your joints. These exercises can be done at a pace that feels comfortable to you and gradually increased as you build strength and endurance.

One of the easiest ways to start incorporating cardio into your routine is by walking. Brisk walking is an excellent form of cardiovascular exercise that can be done almost anywhere. Whether it's a quick walk around the block, a stroll through the park, or walking on a treadmill at the gym, walking is an accessible and effective way to improve heart health. Aim for at least 30 minutes of brisk walking most days of the week, but remember that even

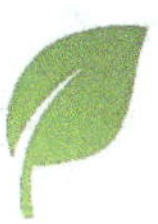

shorter walks are beneficial, and you can gradually increase your time as you feel more comfortable.

Starting with Low-Impact Activities

If walking feels too intense, or if you experience joint pain, consider low-impact alternatives like swimming or water aerobics. The buoyancy of the water supports your body, reducing strain on your joints while providing an excellent cardio workout. Swimming laps or simply walking in the water can improve cardiovascular health, build muscle, and increase flexibility without putting excess pressure on the body. Many seniors also enjoy water aerobics classes, which combine gentle movements with cardio, making it both fun and effective.

Cycling, either outdoors or on a stationary bike, is another low-impact option that can improve heart health while building leg strength. Cycling can be done at a comfortable pace and is easy on the knees and hips, making it an ideal choice for women who may have joint issues. Just like with walking, aim for consistency. Starting with 10 to 15 minutes per session and gradually increasing your time can lead to significant health improvements.

Consistency and Enjoyment Are Key

The most important aspect of cardiovascular exercise is consistency. It's not about doing intense workouts every day; it's about incorporating some form of cardio regularly into your routine. Whether you're walking, swimming, cycling, or dancing, find a form of cardio that you enjoy, so it becomes a habit. You don't have to do it all at once— small, frequent sessions throughout the week add up and provide substantial heart-healthy benefits.

As you continue to exercise regularly, you'll likely notice improvements in your stamina, energy levels, and overall well-being. Your heart will grow stronger, and everyday tasks will feel easier. Plus, regular cardio exercise can help you manage your weight, reduce stress, and promote better sleep, all of which contribute to an enhanced quality of life.

Incorporating cardiovascular exercises into your routine is an essential part of staying healthy and active as you age. You don't need to be a marathon runner to experience the benefits—just start with activities that are easy, enjoyable, and sustainable, and gradually increase your activity level as you feel stronger. Your heart, and your overall health, will thank you for it.

3.3 Strength Training Basics with and Without Weights

Strength training is an incredibly important component of any fitness routine, especially for women over 60. As we age, we naturally lose muscle mass—a condition known as sarcopenia—which can lead to weakness, decreased mobility, and an increased risk of falls and fractures. But the good news is that strength training can slow, stop, and even reverse this process. With consistent effort, it helps maintain and build muscle, keeps bones strong, improves balance, and boosts metabolism.

Strength training doesn't always require heavy weights. For beginners or those looking for low-impact options, bodyweight exercises can be just as effective. Movements like squats, lunges, and wall push-ups can strengthen your muscles and improve your functional strength—the type of strength that helps with daily tasks like getting up

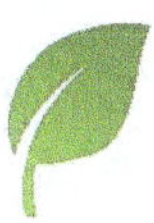

from a chair, carrying groceries, or picking up objects from the floor.

If you're comfortable using weights, starting with light dumbbells or resistance bands can help you further build strength and add variety to your routine. Light hand weights—generally between 1 and 5 pounds—are perfect for beginners and seniors looking to improve strength without straining muscles or joints. For example, using a pair of light weights, you can perform exercises like bicep curls, shoulder presses, and tricep extensions, all of which work key muscles in the arms and shoulders.

Starting with Bodyweight Exercises

Bodyweight exercises are an excellent starting point for seniors because they rely on your own body's weight as resistance, eliminating the need for equipment. These exercises can be modified to suit any fitness level, making them a great option if you're new to strength training. Begin with basic movements that target the lower body, like squats and lunges, or focus on the upper body with wall push-ups or modified push-ups on your knees.

Squats, for example, help build strength in the legs and hips, which are essential for everyday activities such as walking, climbing stairs, and standing up from a seated position. To perform a squat, stand with your feet shoulder-width apart, bend your knees as if you're sitting in a chair, and lower your body while keeping your chest up and your knees behind your toes. Slowly return to standing. You can hold onto a chair or countertop for balance if needed. Start with 10 to 12 repetitions, and as your strength improves, increase the number or add weights.

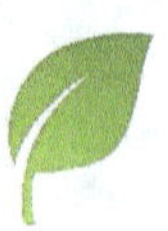

Wall push-ups are a great way to build upper body strength without the strain of full push-ups. Stand facing a wall, place your hands on it slightly wider than shoulder-width apart, and lower your body toward the wall by bending your elbows. Push back to the starting position. This exercise targets the chest, shoulders, and triceps and can be modified by adjusting the angle of your body. As you build strength, you can progress to knee push-ups or full push-ups if desired.

Once you feel comfortable with bodyweight exercises, you can gradually incorporate weights into your strength training routine. Start with light dumbbells or resistance bands and increase the weight as your strength improves. Aim for 2 to 3 strength training sessions per week, allowing at least one rest day between sessions for muscle recovery.

Some key exercises with weights include bicep curls, where you hold a dumbbell in each hand and curl them up toward your shoulders, and shoulder presses, where you lift weights overhead to strengthen the shoulders and arms. For your lower body, you can add weights to your squats or lunges to increase resistance and build strength in the legs and glutes.

It's important to listen to your body while strength training. If an exercise feels too difficult or causes discomfort, it's okay to back off, adjust your form, or decrease the weight. The goal is steady progress, not perfection. Celebrate every increase in strength, no matter how small, and be proud of each workout that brings you closer to your fitness goals.

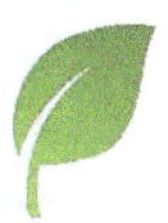

Strength training is a powerful tool for improving your quality of life and maintaining your independence. It's not about lifting heavy weights or achieving a certain look— it's about building a foundation of strength that allows you to move confidently, feel capable, and stay active in the activities you love. Whether you start with bodyweight exercises or gradually incorporate weights, remember that every bit of effort counts toward a healthier, stronger you.

3.4 Balance and Stability Workouts

As we age, maintaining balance and stability becomes crucial for overall health and independence. A fall, even a minor one, can have serious consequences for older adults. But the good news is that balance is something we can improve with regular practice. By incorporating balance exercises into your fitness routine, you can enhance your stability, reduce the risk of falls, and move through your day with greater confidence.

Balance exercises are designed to strengthen the muscles that help keep you upright, as well as improve coordination and flexibility. Simple movements, such as standing on one leg or walking heel-to-toe, can go a long way in building the strength and stability you need to feel secure in your daily activities.

One of the simplest and most effective balance exercises is the **single-leg stand**. Begin by standing behind a sturdy chair or countertop, holding on for support. Lift one leg off the ground and hold the position for 10 to 15 seconds. Switch legs and repeat. As you become more comfortable with this, you can challenge yourself by increasing the time you hold the position or by trying the exercise without holding onto support. If you want to make it even more

challenging, you can close your eyes while balancing. This will help engage your core and improve proprioception—the body's awareness of where it is in space.

Another excellent balance exercise is the **heel-to-toe walk**. This exercise simulates the walking pattern that helps maintain stability when walking in everyday life. Start by standing tall with your feet together. Take a step forward, placing your heel directly in front of your toes (as if walking on a tightrope), and then repeat with the other foot. Continue this for 10 steps, and if you feel confident, try doing it without holding onto a wall or chair for support. This exercise challenges your balance and helps improve coordination.

If standing for extended periods is difficult, there are plenty of balance exercises you can do while seated. Seated marches are a great way to engage the core and improve balance while seated. Sit at the edge of a sturdy chair, with your feet flat on the floor and your back straight. Lift one knee towards your chest, hold for a moment, then lower it back down. Alternate legs in a marching motion. This simple exercise activates the core and hip flexors, which are key to maintaining balance and stability.

Another great seated exercise for improving balance is the **seated leg lift**. While sitting on a chair, extend one leg out in front of you, hold for a few seconds, then lower it back down. Repeat with the other leg. This exercise targets the hip flexors, quadriceps, and core muscles, all of which are important for stabilizing the body and maintaining balance.

As your balance improves, you can add variety and challenge to your routine. For example, you can perform balance exercises while holding light weights or resistance

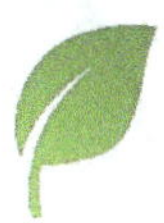

bands to engage your muscles further. Try incorporating these exercises into your daily routine, even if it's just for a few minutes each day. Consistency is key to improving your balance and stability over time.

Balance exercises also offer benefits beyond fall prevention. They help improve posture, increase strength in the legs and core, and promote better body awareness. As you feel more confident in your balance, you may notice that everyday activities—like getting in and out of a car, walking on uneven ground, or standing for longer periods—become easier and more comfortable.

Remember, balance is a skill that improves with practice. Start with simple exercises, listen to your body, and gradually increase the difficulty as you become stronger and more stable. The goal is not perfection but progress. Every small step toward better balance adds up, helping you stay active, independent, and confident in your everyday movements.

3.5 Chair Exercises for Limited Mobility

Chair exercises are a fantastic way for seniors with limited mobility to stay active and improve strength, flexibility, and overall health. Whether you're recovering from an injury, managing a chronic condition, or simply prefer exercises that don't require standing, chair exercises allow you to get moving in a safe and comfortable way. They provide the benefits of a full-body workout without putting unnecessary strain on your joints, and they can be easily modified to suit your personal needs.

Chair exercises often start with upper body movements, which are a great way to build strength and improve

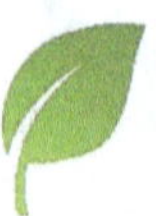

posture. One simple exercise is the **seated shoulder press**. Sit tall in a chair with your feet flat on the floor and a weight in each hand (you can use light hand weights, or even household items like water bottles). Raise your arms to shoulder height and then press the weights overhead, straightening your arms. Lower the weights back to shoulder height and repeat for 10-12 repetitions. This exercise works the shoulders, arms, and upper back, helping to improve posture and reduce stiffness.

Another great upper body exercise is the **seated row**, which strengthens the upper back, shoulders, and arms. Sit upright with your feet flat on the floor and a resistance band in front of you. Hold the band with both hands and stretch it across your body, pulling your elbows back as if you're rowing a boat. Squeeze your shoulder blades together as you pull, and slowly return to the starting position. Aim for 10-12 repetitions. This exercise helps improve posture and can reduce tension in the upper back, which is common when sitting for long periods.

Strengthening your core is essential for stability and mobility. Chair exercises can target the abdominal muscles, which are key to maintaining balance and performing everyday activities with ease. One effective core exercise is the **seated knee lift**. Sit tall in your chair with your feet flat on the floor. Lift one knee towards your chest, hold for a moment, and then lower it back down. Alternate between legs for 10-12 repetitions per side. This movement works the lower abs and helps to improve balance by engaging the core.

For lower body strength, the **seated leg extension** is an excellent exercise that targets the quadriceps and improves knee stability. Sit tall with your feet flat on the

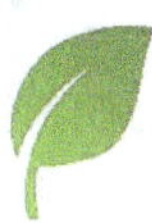

floor. Slowly extend one leg out in front of you, hold for a moment, then lower it back down. Repeat on the other leg. Perform 10-12 repetitions per leg. This exercise helps to improve leg strength and range of motion, which are important for activities like walking and standing up from a chair.

Chair exercises are also excellent for improving flexibility and maintaining a good range of motion. Gentle stretches can help alleviate stiffness and improve circulation. One great stretch is the **seated forward bend**. Sit tall with your feet flat on the floor and slowly bend forward from the hips, reaching toward your toes. Hold the stretch for 15-30 seconds, then slowly return to an upright position. This stretch targets the hamstrings, lower back, and hips, helping to improve flexibility and ease tightness.

Another useful stretch is the **seated spinal twist**, which helps improve flexibility in the spine and can alleviate back discomfort. Sit tall with your feet flat on the floor. Place one hand on the back of the chair and gently twist your torso towards that side. Hold for 15-30 seconds, then return to the center and repeat on the other side. This stretch helps improve mobility in the back and can promote better posture.

Creating a Chair Exercise Routine

You can create a complete workout routine using chair exercises by combining strength, balance, and flexibility moves. Aim to perform a series of exercises, focusing on different muscle groups for 10-15 minutes each day. The key is consistency—incorporating chair exercises into your daily routine will help you maintain strength, flexibility, and mobility, all while staying comfortable and safe. As

your strength and mobility improve, you can gradually increase the duration or intensity of your workouts.

Chair exercises are an excellent way to stay active, regardless of mobility limitations. They provide a full-body workout that can help improve strength, flexibility, and overall health, all while respecting your body's current needs and limitations. By making chair exercises a regular part of your routine, you'll stay strong, independent, and confident, ready to enjoy life's activities with greater ease and comfort.

CHAPTER 4:

SPECIAL FOCUS EXERCISES

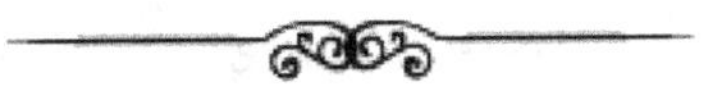

Introduction

In this chapter, we explore special focus exercises tailored for seniors dealing with specific health conditions that impact their mobility and daily life. These exercises are designed to provide relief, enhance mobility, and improve quality of life, while being gentle enough to accommodate various limitations. Whether you're managing arthritis, osteoporosis, recovering from a stroke, or seeking to alleviate back pain, this chapter offers carefully selected exercises to meet your needs. Each exercise will be explained in detail, ensuring you can perform them safely and effectively to gain the most benefit.

4.1 Exercises Tailored for Arthritis Sufferers

Objective: Enhance joint flexibility, reduce pain, and improve daily functional movements.

Warm-up: Gentle Joint Rotations

- Start by sitting comfortably in a chair with your feet flat on the ground.

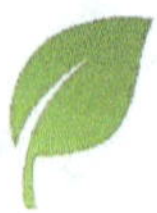

- Slowly rotate your wrists clockwise and then counterclockwise for 10 repetitions each.

- Move to your ankles, rotating them in the same manner to promote synovial fluid movement around the joints.

Strengthening Exercises: Squeeze Ball

- Hold a soft tennis ball or a similar sized stress ball in one hand.

- Gently squeeze the ball and hold for 3-5 seconds, then release.

- Repeat 10 times for each hand.

- This exercise helps strengthen your grip while being gentle on your finger joints.

Flexibility Exercises: Water Aerobics

- Participate in a water aerobics class or simply walk in the shallow end of a pool.

- Use smooth, controlled movements to walk through the water, which provides resistance without the impact.

- Aim for 15-20 minutes, focusing on moving different joints gently through their range of motion.

4.2 Low-Impact Workouts for Osteoporosis Prevention

Objective: Build bone density and maintain bone health through strength training and weight-bearing activities.

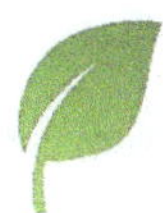

Resistance Training: Resistance Bands

- Sit or stand with good posture and a resistance band under your feet.

- Hold the ends of the band with both hands, arms by your sides.

- Slowly pull the bands upwards while bending your elbows, then lower them back down.

- Perform 10-12 repetitions, ensuring that movements are slow and controlled.

Weight-Bearing Exercises: Gentle Step Aerobics

- Using a low aerobic step or the bottom step of a staircase, step up with one foot, followed by the other, then step down in reverse order.

- Continue for 10-15 minutes at a pace that feels comfortable.

- This exercise promotes bone strength by using your body weight as resistance.

4.3 Hand and Finger Exercises to Improve Dexterity

Objective: Improve fine motor skills and hand strength, enhancing the ability to perform everyday tasks.

Dexterity Drills: Clay Modeling

- Use a small amount of modeling clay or playdough.

- Roll, pinch, and squeeze the clay in various ways to manipulate it into different shapes.

- Spend 10-15 minutes daily on this activity to strengthen hand muscles and improve dexterity.

Fine Motor Skills: Bead Stringing

- Prepare a bowl of large beads and a string or shoelace.

- String the beads onto the lace, focusing on using only your fingertips to pick up each bead.

- This activity not only improves coordination but also helps in maintaining joint flexibility in the hands.

4.4 Post-Stroke Recovery Exercises

Objective: Aid recovery by improving coordination, balance, and rebuilding muscle strength.

Coordination Exercises: Tai Chi

- Join a beginner Tai Chi class or follow an online video.

- Focus on performing each movement slowly and with precision, paying attention to your body's balance and posture.

- Practice for 20-30 minutes, gradually increasing complexity as your coordination improves.

Muscle Strength Exercises: Graduated Light Weights

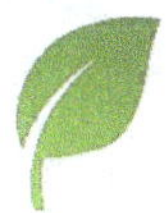

- Start with very light weights (1-2 pounds).

- Perform simple arm raises to the front and side, 10 repetitions each.

- As strength improves, gradually increase the weight and variety of exercises.

4.5 Managing Back Pain Through Exercise

Objective: Strengthen the core and lower back, reducing pain and improving support for the spine.

Core Strengthening: Pelvic Tilts

- Lie on your back with your knees bent and feet flat on the floor.

- Tighten your abdominal muscles and tilt your pelvis towards your chest, flattening your back against the floor.

- Hold for 3-5 seconds, then relax. Repeat 10 times.

Stretching: Gentle Yoga

- Participate in a gentle yoga class focusing on poses that stretch and strengthen the back.

- Poses like Cat-Cow, where you alternate arching and rounding your back, help to increase flexibility and relieve tension in the spine.

- Aim for a 15-20 minute session, focusing on smooth, controlled movements.

CHAPTER 5

DAILY ROUTINES AND CHALLENGES

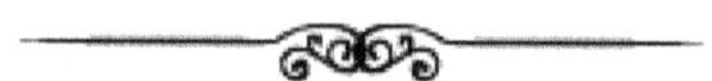

5.1 Creating a Daily Exercise Routine

Introduction

Establishing a daily exercise routine is essential for maintaining health and independence as we age. Consistency is key, and a routine that fits seamlessly into your everyday life can significantly enhance your physical fitness and overall well-being. This section outlines a structured approach to building a manageable daily exercise routine that caters to varying fitness levels and health needs of seniors.

Setting Up Your Daily Routine

Step 1: Define Your Goals

- Start by identifying what you hope to achieve with your exercise routine. Whether it's improving flexibility, building strength, enhancing cardiovascular health, or maintaining balance, your goals will guide the structure of your routine.

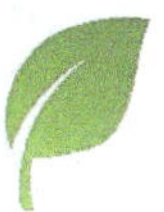

Step 2: Assess Your Current Fitness Level

- Understanding your current fitness level is crucial. This assessment will help tailor the intensity and type of exercises in your routine, ensuring they are both safe and effective.

Step 3: Plan Your Exercise Components

- **Flexibility Exercises**: Begin your day with flexibility exercises to warm up your muscles and joints. Morning stretching can include movements like neck rolls, arm stretches, and leg stretches, which help reduce stiffness and increase mobility.

- **Cardiovascular Activity**: Incorporate at least 30 minutes of cardiovascular activity. This could be a brisk walk in the morning or a session on a stationary bike. If 30 minutes at once is too demanding, break it into shorter sessions—such as three 10-minute walks throughout the day.

- **Strength Training**: Engage in strength training exercises at least two days a week. Use light weights, resistance bands, or body-weight exercises like squats and wall push-ups to maintain muscle mass and support bone health.

- **Balance Exercises**: Balance exercises are crucial for preventing falls. Include balance-focused activities like standing on one leg or heel-to-toe walking at least once a day.

Step 4: Schedule Your Exercises

- **Consistent Timing**: Try to schedule your exercise sessions at the same time each day to establish a routine. For instance, stretching in the morning, a walk after lunch, and strength training in the evening.

- **Flexibility in Scheduling**: While consistency is important, flexibility allows you to adjust based on how you feel on a given day. Listen to your body—if you need a lighter exercise day, adjust accordingly.

Step 5: Monitor and Adjust

- Regularly assess how the routine fits with your lifestyle and physical response. Adjust the intensity, duration, or type of exercises based on your progress and any health changes.

Creating a Supportive Environment

- Ensure that your exercise environment is safe and inviting. Keep any necessary equipment like mats, resistance bands, or weights easily accessible and in good condition.

- Consider the social aspect of exercise. Engaging with friends or groups, even virtually, can provide motivation and accountability.

Conclusion

A well-structured daily exercise routine not only improves physical health but also enhances mental well-being, providing a sense of achievement and routine. By following these steps, seniors can create a sustainable

and enjoyable exercise habit that enhances their quality of life and maintains their independence. This routine can evolve over time as fitness levels improve or as different needs arise, making it a lifelong approach to health and activity.

5.2 30-Day Challenge for Beginners

Week 1: Building a Foundation

Day 1: Morning Stretch Routine

- **Exercise**: Neck Rolls

- **How to Do It**: Sit or stand comfortably. Gently lower your chin to your chest, then slowly roll your head clockwise in a full circle. Do three circles, then switch to counterclockwise.

- **Benefits**: Reduces neck stiffness, enhances flexibility.

Day 2: Morning Stretch Routine, Continued

- **Exercise**: Arm Stretches

- **How to Do It**: Extend one arm overhead, bend the elbow to reach down your back. Use your other hand to gently press the bent elbow for a deeper stretch. Hold for 15 seconds, then switch arms.

- Benefits: Stretches the triceps and shoulders, improving upper body mobility.

Day 3: Morning Stretch Routine, Add Leg Stretches

- **Exercise**: Seated Hamstring Stretch

- **How to Do It**: Sit on the edge of a chair, extend one leg out straight with the heel on the floor, toes pointed up. Lean forward gently from your hips until you feel a stretch in the back of your thigh. Hold for 15-20 seconds, then switch legs.

- Benefits: Increases flexibility in the hamstrings, enhancing leg mobility.

Day 4: Introduce Walking

- **Activity**: Brisk Walking

- **How to Do It**: Walk at a brisk pace that elevates your heart rate but allows you to speak comfortably. Aim for a 15-minute walk in a safe, flat area.

- **Benefits**: Enhances cardiovascular health, boosts mood and energy.

Day 5: Combine Stretching and Walking

- **Morning**: Repeat the stretch routine from Days 1-3.

- **Afternoon**: 15-minute brisk walk, focusing on maintaining a steady pace.

Day 6: Add Upper Body Stretches

- **Exercise**: Shoulder Shrugs

- **How to Do It**: Sit or stand with your arms at your sides. Lift your shoulders up towards your ears, hold for three seconds, and then release. Repeat 10 times.

- **Benefits**: Relieves tension in the shoulders and neck, promotes relaxation.

Day 7: Review and Rest

- **Activity**: Gentle Stretching

- **Review all the stretches from the week, performing each one gently.**

- **Benefits**: Consolidates the week's learning, allows the body to rest and adapt.

Week 2: Introduction to Strength and Balance

Day 8: Introduce Chair Exercises

- **Exercise**: Seated Leg Extensions

- **How to Do It**: Sit in a chair with your feet flat on the floor. Slowly extend one leg in front of you until it is horizontal. Hold for a second, then lower it back down without letting it touch the floor between repetitions. Perform 10 reps, then switch legs.

- **Benefits**: Strengthens the quadriceps, enhances knee joint stability.

Day 9: Introduce Arm Curls

- **Exercise**: Seated Arm Curls

- **How to Do It**: Sit in a chair with a light weight in each hand, palms facing forward. Curl the weights towards your shoulders by bending your elbows. Lower them back down slowly. Perform 10-12 repetitions.

- **Benefits**: Builds bicep strength and forearm flexibility.

Day 10: Balance Exercise

- **Exercise**: Single-Leg Stand

- **How to Do It**: Stand behind a chair and hold onto the back for support. Lift one foot off the ground, hold the position for up to 10 seconds, then switch feet. Repeat 5 times per leg.

- **Benefits**: Improves balance, strengthens leg muscles, enhances focus.

Day 11-14: Continue alternating between these new exercises, gradually increasing repetitions and holding times as comfortable. Introduce walking on slightly uneven surfaces (like a park path) to challenge your balance further.

Day 15: Increase Walking Duration

- **Activity**: Brisk Walking

- **How to Do It**: Walk at a brisk pace for 20 minutes in a safe area. Focus on maintaining a steady pace.

- **Benefits**: Increases cardiovascular endurance and leg strength.

Day 16: Introduce Gentle Squats

- **Exercise**: Chair Squats

- **How to Do It**: Stand in front of a chair with feet shoulder-width apart. Slowly bend your knees and lower yourself as if to sit, then stop just before touching the chair and stand back up. Perform 10 repetitions.

- **Benefits**: Strengthens thighs, buttocks, and core.

Day 17: Add Simple Balance Moves

- **Exercise**: Heel-to-Toe Walk

- **How to Do It**: Walk in a straight line placing the heel of one foot just in front of the toes of the other foot each time you step. Aim to walk 20 steps in this manner.

- **Benefits**: Improves balance and coordination.

Day 18: Increase Strength Training

- **Exercise**: Wall Push-ups

- **How to Do It**: Stand an arm's length from a wall. Place your hands on the wall at shoulder height and width. Bend your elbows and lower your chest to the wall, then push back to the starting position. Perform 10-12 repetitions.

- **Benefits**: Strengthens the chest, shoulders, and arms without straining the back.

Day 19: Integrate Flexibility and Strength

- **Morning Routine**: Repeat the full stretch routine from Week 1 and add wall push-ups at the end.

Day 20: Active Rest Day

- **Activity**: Light Walking and Stretching

- **How to Do It**: Take a leisurely 15-minute walk, then spend 10 minutes stretching.

- **Benefits**: Promotes recovery while keeping the body active.

Day 21: Review and Intensify

- **Activity**: Perform each exercise introduced in Week 3 with added repetitions or longer duration where possible.

Week 4: Solidifying the Habit

Day 22: Challenge with a Longer Walk

- **Activity**: Brisk Walking

- **How to Do It**: Increase your walk to 25 minutes. Try to include a slight incline if possible, like a gentle hill.

- **Benefits**: Builds stamina and leg strength.

Day 23: Advanced Lower Body Strength

- **Exercise**: Step-ups

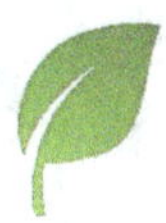

- **How to Do It**: Use a step or a sturdy platform. Step up with one foot, follow with the other, then step down in the reverse order. Perform 10 repetitions on each leg.

- **Benefits**: Enhances leg strength and balance.

Day 24: Enhanced Balance Training

- **Exercise**: Side Leg Raises

- **How to Do It**: Stand behind a chair and hold it for support. Slowly lift one leg to the side, keep it straight, hold for a second, then lower it back down. Perform 10 repetitions on each side.

- **Benefits**: Strengthens hip and outer thigh muscles, improves balance.

Day 25: Full Body Integration

- **Activity**: Combine walking, squats, arm curls, and leg raises in a circuit.

- **How to Do It**: Walk for 5 minutes, perform 10 squats, 10 arm curls with light weights, and 10 side leg raises per leg.

- **Benefits**: Engages the entire body, promoting overall fitness.

Day 26: Stretch and Strengthen

- **Morning Routine**: Engage in a comprehensive stretching session followed by the strength exercises from the previous days.

Day 27: Challenge Your Endurance

- **Activity**: Extend each exercise period by a few minutes or repetitions.

- **How to Do It**: Add 5 minutes to your walking, 2 more repetitions to your squats and push-ups.

- **Benefits**: Pushes your endurance and strength slightly further.

Day 28: Mind and Body Connection

- **Activity**: Practice mindful walking.

- **How to Do It**: Walk for 20 minutes, focusing on each step and breath, maintaining a meditative state.

- **Benefits**: Enhances mental focus, reduces stress, and connects body movements with mental state.

Day 29: Reflect and Plan

- **Activity**: Reflect on the progress made and plan how to incorporate these exercises into a long-term routine.

Day 30: Celebrate and Commit

- **Activity**: Perform a favorite exercise from the challenge, then plan your next month's goals.

- **How to Do It**: Choose an exercise that you particularly enjoyed or benefited from and do it with the intention of celebrating your achievements.

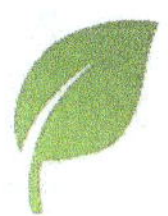

Day 31: Reflective Walk

- **Activity**: Take a leisurely walk in a place you find relaxing, like a park or along a scenic route.

- **How to Do It:** As you walk, think about the physical and mental benefits you've experienced over the past month. Use this time to enjoy the environment and reflect on your journey and future goals.

5.3: Advanced 30-Day Challenge for Active Seniors at Home

This 30-day challenge is designed for active seniors who prefer to exercise at home using minimal equipment like dumbbells or kettlebells. Each day introduces a new exercise that promotes strength, flexibility, balance, and cardiovascular health, ensuring a well-rounded fitness routine.

Week 1: Strength and Flexibility

- **Day 1: Dumbbell Squats**

  - Hold a dumbbell in each hand and perform squats to work the thighs and buttocks.

- **Day 2: Push-Ups**

  - Do a set of push-ups to strengthen the chest, shoulders, and triceps.

- **Day 3: Plank Holds**

  - Hold a plank position to target the core muscles.

- **Day 4: Kettlebell Deadlifts**

  o Use a kettlebell to perform deadlifts, focusing on lower back and hamstring strength.

- **Day 5: Dumbbell Shoulder Press**

  o Press dumbbells overhead to enhance shoulder and upper arm strength.

- **Day 6: Rest Day**

- **Day 7: Review and Reflect**

  o Adjust exercises based on your performance and comfort.

Week 2: Cardio and Core

- **Day 8: High Knees**

  o Run in place lifting your knees high to get your heart rate up.

- **Day 9: Russian Twists**

  o Sit on the floor and twist your torso from side to side holding a dumbbell.

- **Day 10: Burpees**

  o Perform burpees to combine a squat, push-up, and jump into one fluid movement.

- **Day 11: Leg Raises**

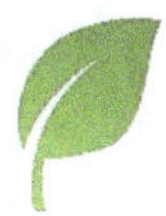

- o Lie on your back and lift your legs to strengthen the lower abdominals.

- **Day 12: Mountain Climbers**

  - o Mimic a climbing motion against the floor to boost cardiovascular endurance.

- **Day 13: Rest Day**

- **Day 14: Reflect and Adjust**

Week 3: Balance and Coordination

- **Day 15: Single-Leg Deadlifts**

  - o Hold a kettlebell in one hand and perform a single-leg deadlift to improve balance and strengthen the hamstrings.

- **Day 16: Side Planks**

  - o Hold a side plank to target the oblique muscles.

- **Day 17: Calf Raises**

  - o Stand on the edge of a step and raise your heels to strengthen the calf muscles.

- **Day 18: Chair Yoga Poses**

  - o Perform a series of yoga poses using a chair for support, focusing on flexibility and balance.

- **Day 19: Toe Touches**

  - o Stand and bend forward trying to touch your toes, to enhance flexibility.

- **Day 20: Rest Day**

- **Day 21: Review and Reflect**

Week 4: Endurance and Strength

- **Day 22: Jogging in Place**

  o Jog in place for a sustained period to build endurance.

- **Day 23: Plank to Push-Up**

  o Start in a plank and move into a push-up position as part of one fluid movement.

- **Day 24: Dumbbell Rows**

  o Bend over slightly and pull dumbbells towards your chest to work the back muscles.

- **Day 25: Squat and Press**

  o Combine a squat with an overhead press using dumbbells for a full-body workout.

- **Day 26: Yoga Flow**

  o Perform a series of yoga movements to improve flexibility and calm the mind.

- **Day 27: Rest Day**

- **Day 28: Reflect and Plan for Continuation**

This tailored 30-day challenge enables more athletic seniors to engage in a dynamic and comprehensive fitness program from the comfort of their homes, utilizing

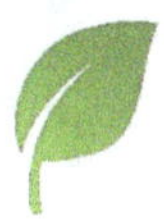

simple equipment. Always focus on maintaining proper form to maximize benefits and minimize the risk of injury.

5.4 Seasonal Exercise Adaptations

Adapting your exercise routine to align with the changing seasons is crucial for maintaining consistency in your fitness journey throughout the year. Seasonal adaptations help cater to the varying environmental conditions, keeping your activities safe, enjoyable, and effective. This section guides seniors on how to modify their routines for different weather conditions and leverage the unique opportunities each season offers.

Spring and Summer: Embrace the Outdoors

Objective: Take advantage of the warmer weather to incorporate more outdoor activities.

Activities:

- **Walking and Hiking**: Increase the duration and complexity of your walks. Explore nature trails which offer both a physical challenge and mental relaxation.

- **Gardening**: Engage in gardening for a soothing yet physically active pastime that enhances your flexibility and endurance.

- **Outdoor Classes**: Participate in outdoor group classes like Tai Chi or water aerobics in a community pool.

How to Adapt:

- **Stay Hydrated**: Increase water intake to compensate for increased perspiration.

- **Wear Appropriate Clothing**: Opt for light-colored, breathable fabrics to stay cool.

- **Time Your Exercises**: Prefer early morning or late evening sessions to avoid peak sun hours.

Fall and Winter: Stay Active Indoors

Objective: Transition to indoor activities that keep you active when the weather cools down.

Activities:

- **Indoor Swimming**: Use indoor pools to continue water aerobics or lap swimming.

- **Mall Walking**: Walk in local malls for a safe, temperature-controlled environment.

- **Home Workouts**: Utilize home exercise videos or equipment for strength training and cardio.

How to Adapt:

- **Layer Up**: Dress in layers to adjust easily to varying indoor temperatures.

- **Create a Home Gym Space**: Set up a dedicated area in your home where you can exercise comfortably.

- **Socialize**: Join indoor classes or groups to keep the social aspect of exercise, which can be motivating during shorter, colder days.

Seasonal Tips and Precautions

For All Seasons:

- **Regular Review**: Assess your physical condition and the suitability of your activities each season. Adapt the intensity and type of exercises based on your current health status.

- **Prevent Seasonal Affective Disorder (SAD)**: Stay active to help manage symptoms of SAD during the winter months by engaging in exercises that boost endorphin levels.

Special Considerations:

- **Fall Risk in Autumn and Winter**: Be cautious of slippery conditions due to wet leaves or ice. Choose footwear with good traction and remain vigilant while walking outdoors.

- **Heat Exhaustion in Summer**: Recognize signs of heat exhaustion, including excessive sweating, faintness, and muscle cramps. If these symptoms occur, stop exercising immediately and seek a cooler environment.

Seasonal exercise adaptations are not just about continuing your fitness regime year-round; they are about maximizing the benefits of each season while ensuring safety and enjoyment. By planning and adjusting your activities according to the season, you maintain a dynamic and responsive approach to fitness that keeps your body challenged and your mind engaged, no matter the weather outside.

CHAPTE 6:

CHAIR YOGA FOR SENIORS

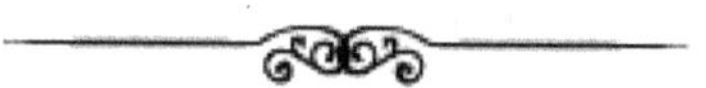

Chair yoga is a wonderful, gentle way to experience the many benefits of yoga without needing to get down on a mat. It's perfect for seniors or anyone who may have mobility issues, providing support and stability while still allowing for a wide range of movement. Chair yoga helps increase flexibility, improve balance, reduce stress, and enhance overall well-being—all from the comfort and safety of a chair. In this chapter, we'll walk through a detailed, step-by-step guide to some chair yoga exercises that you can incorporate into your daily routine.

Remember, these exercises should feel comfortable and enjoyable. Take your time, breathe deeply, and listen to your body. The goal is not to push your limits, but to gently stretch and strengthen in a way that feels right for you.

6.1 Benefits of Chair Yoga

Chair yoga offers many of the same benefits as traditional yoga, including:

- **Improved flexibility**: Helps maintain the range of motion in joints, reducing stiffness.

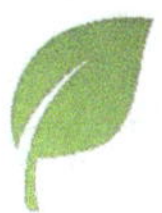

- **Better balance**: Builds muscle strength and stability, which helps prevent falls.

- **Stress reduction**: Calming breathing and mindful movements reduce stress and enhance relaxation.

- **Enhanced circulation**: Gentle movement increases blood flow, supporting overall health.

- **Mental clarity**: Focusing on the breath and gentle poses helps improve concentration and cognitive function.

6.2 Chair Yoga Exercises

1. Seated Mountain Pose (Tadasana)

This pose is a grounding posture that helps establish balance and stability in the body.

- **Step-by-Step**:

  1. Sit up straight with your feet flat on the floor, hip-width apart.

  2. Place your hands on your thighs or let them rest by your sides.

  3. Press your feet firmly into the floor and engage your leg muscles.

  4. Lengthen your spine, lifting the crown of your head towards the ceiling.

5. Take deep breaths, feeling the connection to the ground through your feet and the length in your spine.

• **Benefits**: Improves posture, strengthens core and leg muscles, and promotes a sense of grounding and stability.

2. Seated Forward Bend (Uttanasana)

This gentle forward bend stretches the back, shoulders, and legs, releasing tension and improving flexibility.

• **Step-by-Step**:

1. Sit on the edge of your chair with your feet flat on the floor.

2. Inhale deeply, then exhale as you slowly bend forward from your hips.

3. Let your hands slide down your legs, reaching towards your feet.

4. Allow your head and neck to relax, and breathe deeply.

5. Hold for 3-5 breaths, then slowly roll back up to a seated position.

• **Benefits**: Stretches the spine and hamstrings, releases tension in the back, and improves flexibility.

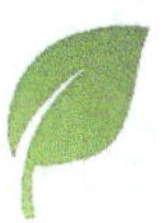

3. Seated Cat-Cow Stretch (Marjaryasana-Bitilasana)

This movement sequence helps to improve flexibility in the spine, relieve back pain, and promote gentle movement in the torso.

- **Step-by-Step**:

    1. Sit up tall with your hands on your knees and feet flat on the floor.

    2. Inhale as you arch your back, lifting your chest and tilting your pelvis forward (Cow Pose).

    3. Exhale as you round your back, pulling your belly button towards your spine and tucking your chin (Cat Pose).

    4. Continue to move with your breath, alternating between Cat and Cow for 5-8 breaths.

- **Benefits**: Improves spine flexibility, reduces stiffness, and increases mobility in the back and neck.

4. Seated Twist (Ardha Matsyendrasana)

Twisting postures help to stretch the back, massage the abdominal organs, and improve digestion.

- **Step-by-Step**:

    1. Sit sideways on the chair with your feet flat on the floor.

    2. Place your hands on the back of the chair.

3.   Inhale, lengthen your spine, and on the exhale, gently twist your torso towards the back of the chair.

4.   Keep your back straight and avoid straining.

5.   Hold for 3-5 breaths, then release and switch sides.

•   **Benefits**: Stretches the spine, improves digestion, and enhances flexibility in the back.

5. Seated Warrior Pose (Virabhadrasana)

A modified version of the traditional standing Warrior pose, this posture strengthens the legs and core and promotes a sense of empowerment.

•   **Step-by-Step**:

1.   Sit sideways on the chair with your right leg extended out to the side.

2.   Bend your left knee at a 90-degree angle, with your foot flat on the floor.

3.   Raise your arms parallel to the floor, reaching them out in opposite directions.

4.   Hold for 3-5 breaths, feeling the strength in your legs and arms.

5.   Switch sides and repeat.

•   **Benefits**: Strengthens the legs, improves balance, and enhances core stability.

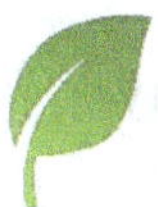

6. Seated Eagle Pose (Garudasana)

This pose opens the shoulders, improves focus, and stretches the arms and upper back.

- **Step-by-Step**:

  1. Sit up straight with your feet flat on the floor.

  2. Extend your arms in front of you and cross your right arm over your left at the elbows.

  3. Bend your elbows and bring your palms together if possible.

  4. Lift your elbows slightly, feeling a stretch in the shoulders.

  5. Hold for 3-5 breaths, then release and switch sides.

- **Benefits**: Increases shoulder flexibility, improves focus, and relieves tension in the upper back.

7. Seated Side Stretch (Parsva Urdhva Hastasana)

This side stretch lengthens the spine and opens up the rib cage, helping to deepen the breath and stretch the sides of the body.

- **Step-by-Step**:

  1. Sit up tall with your feet flat on the floor.

  2. Inhale, lift your right arm overhead, reaching towards the ceiling.

3.   Exhale, lean slightly to the left, feeling the stretch along your right side.

4.   Hold for 3-5 breaths, then switch sides.

•   **Benefits**: Stretches the side body, improves flexibility, and encourages deep breathing.

8. Seated Shoulder Rolls

This gentle exercise relieves tension in the shoulders and neck, improving mobility in the upper body.

•   **Step-by-Step**:

1.   Sit comfortably with your feet flat on the floor.

2.   Inhale, lift your shoulders up towards your ears, then exhale as you roll them back and down.

3.   Repeat this movement for 5-8 breaths.

•   **Benefits**: Relieves tension in the shoulders, improves mobility, and promotes relaxation.

9. Seated Forward Bend with Leg Extension

This variation on the forward bend includes a leg extension for an additional stretch in the hamstrings.

•   **Step-by-Step**:

1.   Sit on the edge of the chair and extend your right leg out with the heel on the floor and toes pointing up.

2.   Inhale, sit up tall, and exhale as you gently lean forward, reaching towards your toes.

3.   Hold for 3-5 breaths, feeling the stretch in the hamstrings.

4.   Switch legs and repeat.

•   **Benefits**: Stretches the hamstrings and lower back, increases flexibility, and reduces tension.

10. Seated Relaxation and Breathing

This final pose allows you to relax, reset, and enjoy the benefits of the practice.

•   **Step-by-Step**:

1.   Sit comfortably with your feet flat on the floor, hands resting on your lap.

2.   Close your eyes and take deep, slow breaths, allowing your body to relax with each exhale.

3.   Focus on the sensation of your breath, letting go of any tension or stress.

4.   Stay in this relaxed state for a few minutes.

•   **Benefits**: Promotes relaxation, reduces stress, and calms the mind.

Chair yoga offers a gentle yet powerful way to build strength, flexibility, and mental clarity. These movements can be incorporated easily into your daily routine, providing physical benefits and a sense of calm and mindfulness. Remember, chair yoga is about listening to

your body, moving with intention, and honoring your abilities. With each pose, breathe deeply, move slowly, and enjoy the connection to your body and mind. Here's to a journey of wellness, one seated stretch at a time.

CHAPTER 7:

NUTRITION AND EXERCISE

As we age, the way we fuel our bodies becomes just as important as the exercises we do to stay healthy and active. Good nutrition helps seniors maximize their energy, maintain a healthy weight, and support muscle and bone health. This chapter provides practical, easy-to-follow guidance on nutrition to complement your fitness routine and help you feel your best every day.

7.1 Eating for Energy: Nutrition Tips for Active Seniors

Exercise requires energy, and what we eat directly impacts how energetic and strong we feel. The good news? You don't have to overhaul your entire diet. Small adjustments can make a big difference in how you feel throughout the day.

Focus on Protein

Protein is vital for maintaining muscle mass, which naturally declines with age. Regular exercise helps combat this, but pairing it with enough protein can make a real difference. Good sources of protein include chicken, fish, eggs, beans, tofu, and Greek yogurt. Aim to include

a protein source in each meal, whether it's a handful of nuts in the morning or a piece of grilled fish at dinner.

- **Tip**: Try a "protein snack" after exercise, such as a small serving of cottage cheese or a few slices of turkey. This helps with muscle recovery and keeps energy levels steady.

Embrace Whole Grains

Carbohydrates often get a bad rap, but they're actually a great source of energy—when you choose the right kinds. Whole grains like oats, brown rice, and whole wheat pasta provide a slow and steady energy release. They're rich in fiber, which helps keep you feeling full and supports healthy digestion. So don't shy away from carbs, just reach for whole-grain options that will keep you going without causing spikes in blood sugar.

- **Tip**: Try oatmeal with a sprinkle of nuts and berries for breakfast. It's filling, easy on the stomach, and provides lasting energy.

Load Up on Fruits and Vegetables

Vibrant fruits and vegetables are packed with vitamins, minerals, and antioxidants, which can help reduce inflammation and support recovery after exercise. Leafy greens, berries, carrots, and citrus fruits are excellent choices. Plus, they add color to your plate, which can make meals feel more enjoyable.

- **Tip**: Add a serving of greens to every meal, whether it's spinach in your omelet or a side salad at dinner. Don't worry if you don't love salads—there are plenty of creative ways to get more veggies!

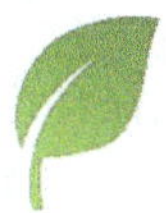

7.2 Hydration: How Much to Drink Before, During, and After Exercise

Staying hydrated is essential for good health and is especially important when exercising. As we age, we may not feel thirsty as often, but that doesn't mean our bodies don't need water.

Before Exercise

Start hydrating early in the day. A good rule of thumb is to drink a glass of water about an hour before you exercise. If it's been a while since you had a drink, have a small glass just before you start, but don't overdo it to avoid feeling bloated.

- **Tip**: If plain water isn't appealing, try adding a slice of lemon or cucumber for a refreshing twist.

During Exercise

For light to moderate activities, sipping water every 15-20 minutes should keep you hydrated. For shorter exercises, you might not need a drink break, but be sure to listen to your body—if you feel thirsty, take a sip.

After Exercise

After exercising, it's essential to rehydrate to replace any fluids you may have lost. A glass or two of water post-exercise is usually enough, especially if your activity was gentle to moderate. If you've had a longer or more intense workout, you may want to drink a bit more.

- **Tip**: A glass of water with a slice of orange or a splash of juice is a great way to replenish electrolytes naturally.

7.3 Supplements: What Helps and What Doesn't

Supplements can be a tricky area, with many options on the market. Some may be beneficial, while others might not be necessary if you're already eating a balanced diet. Here's a guide to a few supplements commonly recommended for seniors:

Calcium and Vitamin D

Calcium is vital for bone health, and vitamin D helps our bodies absorb calcium. As we age, our bones naturally lose density, making these nutrients even more important. If you're not getting enough calcium from foods like dairy, leafy greens, or fortified cereals, a supplement may help. Many seniors also benefit from vitamin D supplements, as it can be hard to get enough from sunlight alone.

Omega-3 Fatty Acids

Omega-3s, found in fatty fish like salmon and mackerel, are great for heart health and can help reduce inflammation. If you're not a big fish eater, consider an omega-3 supplement. Studies suggest omega-3s may also support joint health, which is beneficial for active seniors.

B Vitamins

B vitamins, especially B12, play a role in energy metabolism and nerve health. As we get older, it can become harder for our bodies to absorb B12 from food. If

you're feeling fatigued or your doctor has indicated low B12 levels, a supplement could help.

What to Avoid

While some supplements are beneficial, others may not be necessary and could even interfere with medications or cause side effects. Always consult your healthcare provider before starting any new supplement, especially if it's marketed as a "quick fix" or miracle solution. And remember, there's no replacement for a balanced diet!

Fueling your body with the right foods and ensuring adequate hydration and supplementation can support your exercise routine and overall well-being. While exercise builds strength and vitality, good nutrition provides the fuel to make those workouts effective and enjoyable. The best approach is to keep it simple—focus on whole foods, hydrate, and consult a healthcare provider when considering supplements.

Remember, you're investing in your health with every nutritious choice you make. And hey, if you slip up now and then (we all enjoy a treat!), that's okay. Balance, after all, is about enjoying both the healthy habits and the occasional indulgence along the way. So toast your glass of water (or your favorite smoothie) to the journey ahead, and know that every step you take is one toward a healthier, more vibrant you!

CHAPTER 8:

COMMUNITY AND SOCIAL ENGAGEMENT

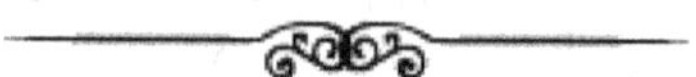

Staying active and healthy is not only about the exercises you do or the food you eat—it's also about the connections you make along the way. For seniors, staying socially engaged can be as vital as staying physically active. Research shows that strong social connections can boost mental health, reduce stress, and even improve physical health outcomes. In this chapter, we explore ways to build a supportive community around your fitness journey, connect with others who share similar goals, and find inspiration from seniors who stay active and embrace life.

8.1 Joining Exercise Groups and Classes

One of the easiest and most rewarding ways to build community is by joining group exercise classes tailored for seniors. Exercising with others not only helps you stay motivated but also adds an element of fun and companionship to your routine. Whether it's a yoga class, water aerobics, or a walking group, there's something special about connecting with others who share similar goals.

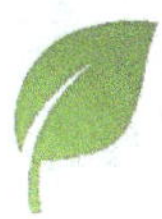

Benefits of Group Exercise

- **Accountability**: When you commit to a group, you're more likely to show up. Regular exercise becomes part of a routine shared by others, so even on days when you're not feeling your best, knowing that others are counting on you can be a big motivator.

- **Social Interaction**: Exercising with others is a fantastic way to socialize. It provides a regular opportunity to catch up with friends, share stories, and build relationships.

- **Support and Encouragement**: In a group setting, everyone is working towards similar goals, and that shared journey can be very encouraging. It's heartening to see others making progress and to have friends to cheer you on when you reach milestones.

Types of Group Classes for Seniors

- **Water Aerobics**: Ideal for those with joint pain or mobility issues, water aerobics is gentle on the body but provides an excellent workout. The water's buoyancy reduces stress on the joints, while the resistance of moving through water builds strength.

- **Yoga and Chair Yoga**: Yoga classes tailored for seniors focus on flexibility, balance, and relaxation. Chair yoga is particularly helpful for those who may need support.

- **Dance Classes**: Dance-based workouts like Zumba Gold (a gentler version of Zumba) are

fantastic for both cardio and coordination. Plus, the music makes it feel like a fun social event!

- **Walking Groups**: Organized walking groups are simple, low-impact, and accessible. They're perfect for those who want a regular, outdoor activity that encourages conversation.

How to Find a Group

Check with your local community center, senior center, or gym to see if they offer classes specifically for seniors. Many centers offer affordable or even free classes tailored for different fitness levels. Libraries, local newspapers, or online platforms like Meetup may also list community exercise groups that welcome seniors.

8.2 Using Technology to Stay Connected with Exercise Partners

Technology has made it easier than ever to connect with others, even if they're not physically nearby. For seniors, using technology to stay engaged with exercise partners can add a new dimension to fitness routines, keeping you motivated and accountable while bridging distances. Here are some practical ways to use technology to stay connected.

Joining an online class or creating a virtual exercise meetup group can help you stay socially connected. Many seniors' classes are now available online, offering everything from chair yoga to Pilates and Tai Chi. With video platforms like Zoom or Google Meet, you can work out with friends, check in with each other, and keep each other motivated.

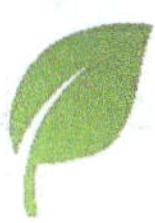

There are several apps designed to make exercise more interactive. Some apps allow you to track your workouts, share progress with friends, and join virtual communities where you can celebrate achievements together.

Example Apps:

- **Fitbit**: Track your daily steps, sleep, and exercise. You can connect with friends, join challenges, and cheer each other on.

- **MyFitnessPal**: A comprehensive app for tracking nutrition and activity. It has social features for sharing goals and connecting with friends.

- **SilverSneakers GO**: Created specifically for seniors, this app includes workout programs, classes, and progress tracking.

Creating a Digital Fitness Network

You don't have to use formal apps to stay connected with friends. A simple group text or chat group on a platform like WhatsApp or Facebook Messenger can keep you in touch with exercise partners. Share updates on your daily walk, swap healthy recipes, or even share a funny story from your workout. Staying connected doesn't have to be complicated—it's about building friendships and sharing encouragement.

8.3 Stories of Inspiration: Seniors Who Stay Active

There's nothing like a little inspiration to remind us of what's possible at any age. Here are some inspiring stories of seniors who have embraced an active lifestyle, showing that age truly is just a number.

Marjorie's Journey with Walking

At 78, Marjorie discovered a love for walking that changed her life. When her doctor recommended more activity to improve her heart health, she started small—just a 10-minute walk around her block each day. Gradually, she built up her stamina, eventually joining a local walking group. Today, Marjorie walks three miles daily, rain or shine, and has made wonderful friends along the way. "I never thought I'd look forward to walking, but it's the best part of my day now," she says with a smile.

Frank's Adventure with Water Aerobics

Frank, a 70-year-old retired firefighter, struggled with arthritis and had almost given up on exercise. But a friend convinced him to try water aerobics at the local YMCA, and it's been a game-changer. "Being in the water feels freeing," Frank says. The support from the water allowed him to move more comfortably, and now he's part of a tight-knit group that meets every week. Frank credits water aerobics with not only improving his flexibility but also introducing him to friends who keep him laughing.

Sophia's Pilates Transformation

At 66, Sophia was looking for an exercise that could improve her posture and reduce back pain. She tried a few classes before discovering Pilates and quickly fell in love with it. The slow, controlled movements helped strengthen her core, and her back pain started to diminish. Today, she attends two classes a week and even practices at home. "I feel stronger than ever," she says, "and I love the sense of balance it brings to my life."

8.4 Tips for Building Your Own Community

Building a fitness community doesn't have to happen all at once. Whether you're looking to join an established group, connect with friends online, or create something new in your neighborhood, here are some practical tips for building a supportive and enjoyable fitness community.

If joining a big class feels overwhelming, start with a friend or family member. Invite a neighbor to join you for a morning walk or ask a friend if they'd like to try a yoga class together. Sometimes the best communities start with just one or two people.

Consistency is key when it comes to building relationships. Set a regular schedule, whether it's a weekly walk, a virtual check-in, or a class you attend every Monday. People are more likely to join and stay engaged when there's a set routine.

As you find enjoyment in your routine, consider inviting others. Your enthusiasm can be contagious, and sometimes people just need a little nudge to get started. Whether it's a new friend from church, a family member, or a fellow library-goer, extend the invitation and see where it leads.

Every milestone, no matter how small, is worth celebrating. Maybe you walked an extra block today or attended a new class. Share these achievements with your group and cheer each other on. Celebrating progress, however small, keeps the energy positive and the motivation strong.

A fitness community is about more than just workouts. Make time to grab a coffee, catch up on life, or simply chat about your week. These connections create a stronger bond, and you'll be more likely to stay engaged when you're invested in each other's lives.

Exercise is about more than just staying fit; it's about staying connected to the people around us and creating a community that uplifts and inspires. A supportive fitness community can bring joy, companionship, and lasting motivation. Whether you're joining an exercise class, forming a walking group, or simply using technology to check in with friends, these connections enrich our lives and make each workout a little more meaningful.

So reach out, join a group, or even start one yourself. Surround yourself with people who share your goals, who cheer you on, and who make the journey enjoyable. After all, life's better with a little company—and a lot of encouragement—along the way.

CHAPTER 9:

MEASURING PROGRESS

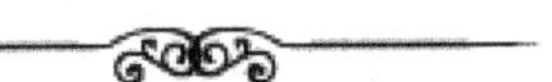

Setting and tracking your progress is a key part of maintaining motivation and achieving long-term success in your fitness journey. It's not only about the physical changes you can see but also about the subtle, positive shifts in strength, balance, energy, and even confidence. This chapter will guide you through setting meaningful goals, tracking your achievements, and adjusting your exercise plan as you progress.

9.1 How to Track Your Exercise Progress

Tracking your progress doesn't have to be complicated. By recording a few key details after each workout or at the end of each week, you can get a clear picture of how far you've come and where you want to go.

Start with a Journal or Log

Using a simple journal or exercise log can be an effective way to track your progress. Write down what exercises you did, how long you did them for, and how you felt afterward. Tracking the "how you feel" part is especially important because progress isn't always about numbers;

it's also about feeling stronger, more energetic, or less stiff.

What to Track:

- **Duration**: How long you spent on each activity.

- **Repetitions**: The number of repetitions (for strength exercises) or laps (for swimming).

- **Intensity**: Note how challenging the exercise felt, using a scale of 1-10.

- **Flexibility and Balance**: For stretching and balance exercises, jot down whether certain poses feel easier or harder over time.

- **Mood and Energy**: This can give insights into how exercise is affecting your well-being.

If you prefer to keep things digital, there are several apps designed for tracking exercise, such as Fitbit, MyFitnessPal, or even a simple notes app on your phone. These tools can track steps, calories burned, exercise duration, and more. Some apps even allow you to connect with friends, giving you a little extra encouragement and accountability.

At the end of each week or month, review your journal or app and look for patterns. Are you able to walk a little farther without getting tired? Have you increased your strength training weights or reps? These check-ins will help you see progress over time, even if it's gradual. Remember, even small improvements are victories worth celebrating!

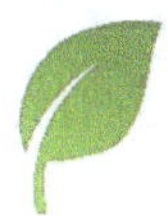

9.2 Setting and Revising Goals

Goals give us something to work toward, and they help keep us focused. The key to setting effective fitness goals is to make them specific, realistic, and personally meaningful.

SMART Goals

A great method for setting goals is to make them SMART: Specific, Measurable, Achievable, Relevant, and Time-bound.

- **Specific**: Instead of saying "I want to get stronger," specify exactly how. For example, "I want to be able to do 10 wall push-ups without stopping."

- **Measurable**: Include a way to measure progress, like distance or repetition. "Walk a mile in 20 minutes" is easier to track than "improve walking."

- **Achievable**: Set goals you can realistically achieve based on your current fitness level.

- **Relevant**: Make sure your goals are meaningful to you. If you love walking outdoors, setting a goal related to walking is more relevant and motivating.

- **Time-bound**: Give yourself a timeline. For example, "By the end of this month, I want to complete a 30-minute walk three times a week."

Examples of SMART Goals:

- "I want to walk for 20 minutes every day for the next two weeks."

- "By the end of the month, I want to increase my seated leg lifts to 20 reps per leg."

- "I will complete three chair yoga sessions each week to improve my flexibility and reduce stiffness."

As you meet your initial goals, it's important to set new ones to keep challenging yourself and to stay motivated. Revisiting your goals every month or two allows you to adjust based on your progress and changing interests. Perhaps you'll decide to focus on balance exercises or work toward lifting slightly heavier weights. Fitness is a journey, and as your abilities evolve, so can your goals.

9.3 When to Update Your Exercise Plan

As you progress, you may find that your current exercise routine no longer feels as challenging or as beneficial as it once did. This is a natural part of improvement, and it's a sign that your body is ready for new challenges. Here's how to recognize when it's time to update your exercise plan.

Signs You're Ready for a New Challenge

- **Exercises Feel Too Easy**: If you're completing your workouts without much effort, it might be time to increase the intensity. For example, if you're doing 10 reps of a strength exercise and barely feeling it, try increasing to 12-15 reps or add a bit more weight.

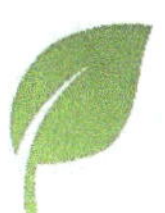

- **You've Plateaued**: Sometimes, progress slows or stalls altogether. If you've been doing the same exercises for months and haven't noticed improvements, mixing things up can help.

- **New Goals or Interests**: As you progress, you may discover new interests. Maybe you'd like to try a new activity, like Pilates, hiking, or ballroom dancing. Updating your routine to align with these interests keeps things fresh and enjoyable.

How to Update Your Plan

1. **Increase Intensity Gradually**: For strength exercises, add a bit more weight, try an extra set, or increase your repetitions. For cardio, add 5-10 minutes to your workout time or try intervals where you pick up the pace for short bursts.

2. **Incorporate New Exercises**: Add new activities that challenge your body in different ways. If you're comfortable with chair exercises, try standing balance poses, or if you've mastered short walks, try including a hill or incline.

3. **Focus on Different Areas**: If you've spent months improving strength, consider shifting focus to flexibility or balance. Rotating focus helps build a well-rounded fitness foundation.

9.4 Celebrating Your Successes

Tracking progress and updating your goals isn't just about improvement—it's about recognizing and celebrating your successes. Celebrating achievements, no matter how

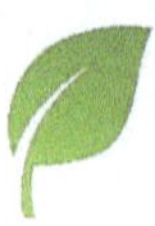

small, keeps you motivated, reinforces positive behavior, and brings joy to your fitness journey.

Celebrating successes—whether it's reaching a goal, increasing your stamina, or simply showing up consistently—reinforces the effort you're putting in. It reminds you of how far you've come and boosts confidence to keep going. A celebration doesn't have to be big, but it should feel rewarding and meaningful to you.

Ideas for Celebrating Successes

- **Treat Yourself**: After reaching a milestone, treat yourself to something special, like a new pair of walking shoes, a fitness tracker, or even a relaxing massage.

- **Share with Friends or Family**: Tell someone close to you about your achievement. They'll likely be thrilled for you, and sharing reinforces the accomplishment.

- **Plan a Fun Outing**: As a reward, plan a day trip or outing. A scenic walk, a visit to a favorite park, or a nice meal can be a wonderful way to enjoy the benefits of your hard work.

- **Document Your Progress**: Take photos or jot down notes on how you felt before versus now. Looking back at this record can be both surprising and rewarding, showing the real impact of your efforts.

Progress isn't always linear, and it's natural to face occasional setbacks. Maybe you miss a week of exercise or feel discouraged if progress is slow. Remember,

setbacks are part of the journey. Every time you get back on track, you're building resilience. So celebrate each time you overcome a setback—returning to your routine is an achievement in itself.

Measuring your progress is about more than numbers on a chart. It's about recognizing your efforts, setting goals that inspire you, and staying motivated through every step of your fitness journey. By setting goals, tracking progress, updating your plan, and celebrating your achievements, you'll stay focused and engaged, making fitness a lasting, enjoyable part of your life.

Every small step you take toward better health adds up over time. Progress might be slow or gradual, but each improvement builds on the last, contributing to a stronger, healthier you. Remember, the journey itself is worth celebrating—so enjoy each step and every achievement along the way. You're investing in your well-being, and there's no better reward than feeling your best and embracing all the possibilities that come with it.

CHAPTER 10:

CONCLUSION

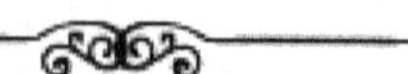

Reaching the end of this guide marks a significant moment in your journey toward a healthier, more active lifestyle. We've covered a wide array of topics, from understanding the benefits of exercise for seniors to creating personalized routines, staying motivated, and building a supportive community. The goal has been to equip you with the tools, knowledge, and encouragement to make exercise a sustainable and enjoyable part of your life.

As you reflect on what you've learned, remember that health and fitness are lifelong journeys. Progress might be gradual, and there will be days when you may feel more challenged than others. But every step you take is a step toward greater strength, resilience, and well-being. This journey is about celebrating what you can achieve, enjoying the movement, and embracing the positive changes you're making for your body and mind.

10.1 Maintaining Motivation Over Time

Motivation can come and go, especially when life gets busy, or energy levels dip. Here are a few strategies to help keep you on track and inspired:

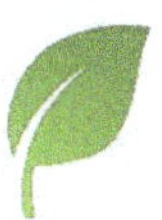

1. **Revisit Your Goals**: Remind yourself of why you started. Whether it's to stay independent, keep up with grandchildren, or improve health, keeping these motivations in mind can fuel your commitment.

2. **Set New Challenges**: As you achieve your initial goals, set new ones to keep things interesting. Maybe it's learning a new form of exercise, increasing your walking distance, or attending a group class regularly.

3. **Celebrate Small Wins**: Don't wait for major milestones to reward yourself. Every day you show up and invest in your health is worth celebrating.

4. **Stay Connected**: Join or maintain your fitness community. Friends, exercise groups, and online connections can provide encouragement and accountability.

5. **Listen to Your Body**: As important as consistency is, it's also crucial to honor how your body feels. Take rest days, adjust intensity when needed, and seek activities that bring joy and comfort, not strain.

Remember, motivation isn't always about feeling excited. Sometimes, it's simply about commitment and showing up for yourself.

10.2 The Long-Term Benefits of Staying Active

Throughout this book, we've touched on many of the benefits that exercise brings to physical, mental, and emotional well-being. But let's look at the big picture—why

staying active is truly one of the best gifts you can give yourself.

1. **Improved Physical Health**: Regular exercise reduces the risk of chronic conditions like heart disease, diabetes, and osteoporosis. It strengthens muscles, supports joint health, and enhances flexibility and balance. This means greater freedom and confidence in daily activities, from grocery shopping to traveling.

2. **Increased Independence**: One of the most valued benefits of fitness for seniors is maintaining independence. Staying physically active can make the difference in being able to perform daily tasks without assistance and staying self-sufficient.

3. **Enhanced Cognitive Function**: Studies show that regular exercise can help protect the brain from age-related decline, improve memory, and boost mood. Physical activity promotes blood flow to the brain, supporting cognition and reducing the risk of depression and anxiety.

4. **Greater Resilience and Adaptability**: As you continue to exercise and improve your fitness, you're building resilience. Physical resilience helps you recover faster from illness or injury, while mental resilience enhances your ability to handle stress and adapt to changes.

5. **Joy and Quality of Life**: Physical fitness enhances every area of life, allowing you to engage fully in activities you love, try new things, and enjoy precious time with family and friends. Staying active

helps create a lifestyle that's vibrant, fulfilling, and rich in experiences.

10.3 Encouragement for Continuing the Journey

Starting and maintaining an exercise routine can feel daunting, but you've already taken the first and most important step by reading this guide and committing to a healthier lifestyle. As you move forward, remember that your journey is unique. It's okay to adapt, try new things, and adjust your routine as you discover what works best for you.

Here are a few final reminders to carry with you:

- **Keep it Fun**: Fitness isn't just about discipline—it's about joy. Find activities that make you feel alive, whether it's dancing, swimming, walking in nature, or practicing yoga. When you enjoy what you're doing, staying active becomes less of a chore and more of a pleasure.

- **Listen to Your Body's Wisdom**: Aging comes with changes, and some days may be harder than others. Let your body guide you in choosing what feels right each day. Respect any limitations and celebrate your strengths.

- **Celebrate the Journey**: Every step, every stretch, and every moment spent moving your body is a victory. Fitness is a journey that's about progress, not perfection. Celebrate your commitment, your perseverance, and the positive changes you're making.

- **Don't Be Afraid to Seek Support**: Remember, you don't have to do it alone. Connect with friends, join a class, or talk to a fitness professional who can provide guidance. Sometimes, a little encouragement or advice is all it takes to renew your motivation.

Final Thoughts

This book is a companion for your journey toward a healthier, more vibrant life. As you embrace fitness and well-being, know that you're doing something remarkable for yourself. Exercise, no matter how gentle or gradual, helps keep you engaged in the world and connected to yourself. It brings a sense of purpose and joy that goes beyond physical health.

Take each day as it comes, approach every workout with a positive mindset, and be kind to yourself on this journey. Every choice you make to move your body, nourish it well, and connect with others is a powerful statement of self-care and self-respect. In a world that can sometimes feel fast-paced and overwhelming, dedicating time to your health is a beautiful reminder that you're taking charge of your future and prioritizing what matters most.

Remember, fitness is for everyone, at every age. Embrace the process, celebrate the progress, and continue to explore new ways to keep moving and growing. Here's to a lifetime of health, happiness, and strength—you deserve every bit of it.

Thank you for allowing this guide to be a part of your journey. Now go out there, stay active, and enjoy every step along the way.

APPENDIX:

DETAILED EXERCISE DESCRIPTIONS

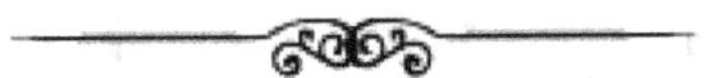

This appendix is carefully curated to provide detailed, step-by-step instructions for each exercise mentioned in the book, ensuring that users can perform each movement safely and effectively. Each entry outlines the steps, benefits, and variations to accommodate different fitness levels, along with safety tips to prevent injury.

1. Arm Circles

- **Steps**:

    1. Stand with your feet shoulder-width apart.

    2. Extend your arms parallel to the floor.

    3. Slowly make small circles with your arms, gradually increasing the diameter.

    4. Continue for 10-15 seconds in one direction, then reverse the direction and repeat.

- **Benefits**: Increases blood circulation and flexibility in the shoulders.

- **Variations**: Increase the size of the circles or adjust the speed.

- **Safety Tips**: Keep the movements smooth to avoid jerking which could strain muscles.

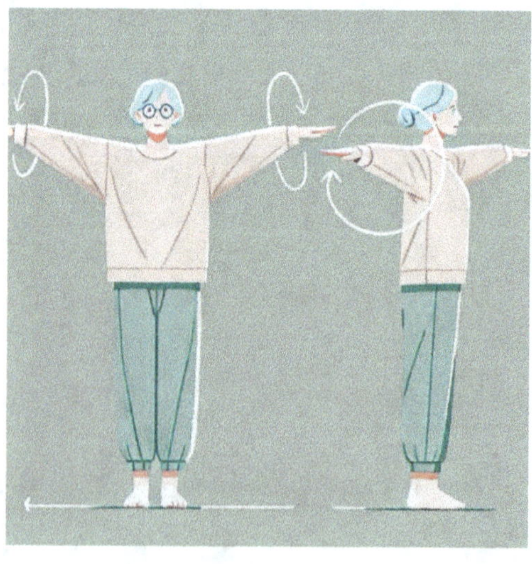

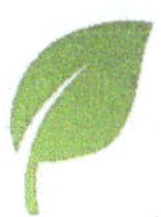

2. Arm Stretches

- **Steps**:

    1. Raise one arm and reach it across your body.

    2. With the opposite hand, gently pull the elbow towards your chest until you feel a stretch in your shoulder and upper arm.

    3. Hold the stretch for 15-20 seconds.

    4. Repeat on the other side.

- **Benefits**: Reduces tension in the upper back and shoulders.

- **Variations**: For a deeper stretch, use a towel or band to hold the stretched arm.

- **Safety Tips**: Do not overstretch or twist the joint uncomfortably.

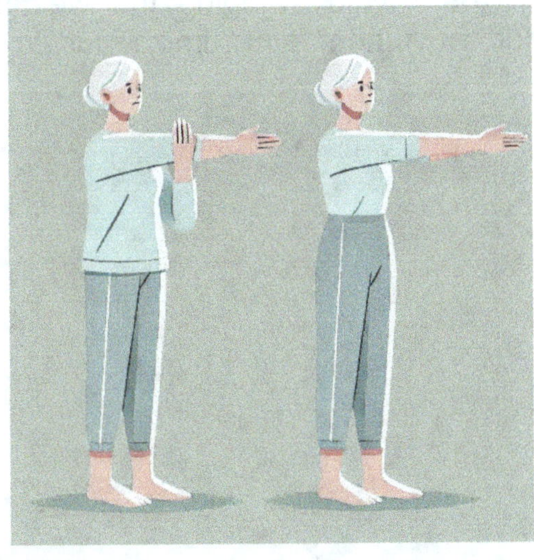

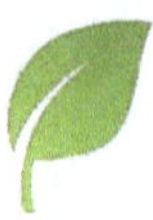

3. Bicep Curls

- **Steps**:

    1. Sit or stand with your feet shoulder-width apart.

    2. Hold a dumbbell in each hand with arms fully extended and palms facing forward.

    3. Curl the weights towards your shoulders by bending your elbows while keeping your upper arms stationary.

    4. Slowly lower the weights back to the starting position.

    5. Repeat for 10-12 repetitions.

- **Benefits**: Strengthens the biceps and improves arm muscle tone.

- **Variations**: Perform alternating curls to focus on each arm individually.

- **Safety Tips**: Avoid swinging the weights; ensure a controlled movement to maximize muscle engagement.

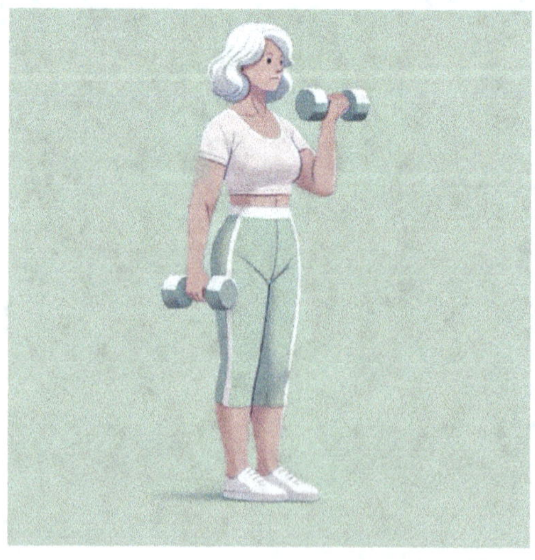

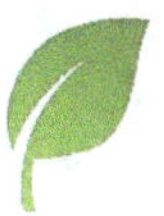

4. Calf Raises

- **Steps**:

    1. Stand upright and support yourself on the back of a chair or against a wall for balance.

    2. Lift your heels off the ground, rising onto your toes.

    3. Hold the peak position for a second before lowering your heels back to the floor.

    4. Perform 10-15 repetitions.

- **Benefits**: Strengthens the calf muscles and improves ankle stability.

- **Variations**: Perform one leg at a time to increase the challenge.

- **Safety Tips**: Rise and lower on a smooth, slow count to avoid balance issues.

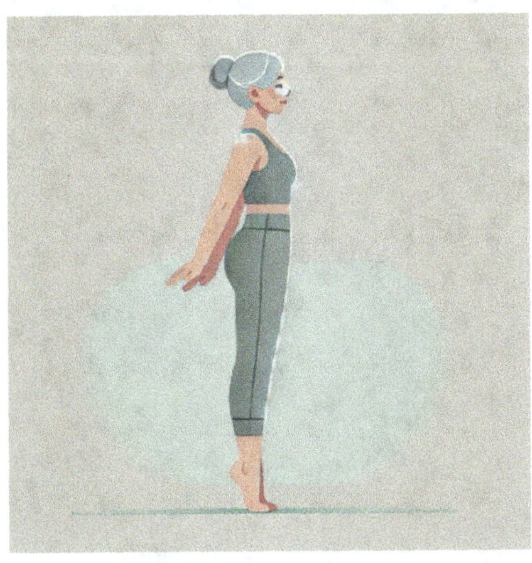

5. Chair Squats

- **Steps**:

    1. Stand in front of a sturdy chair with your feet hip-width apart.

    2. Extend your arms forward for balance if needed.

    3. Slowly bend your knees and lower your hips towards the chair, as if sitting down.

    5. Lightly touch the chair with your buttocks, then stand back up.

    6. Repeat 10-15 times.

- **Benefits**: Enhances leg strength and promotes functional mobility.

- **Variations**: Add a light dumbbell to increase resistance.

- **Safety Tips**: Ensure the chair is stable and does not move during the exercise.

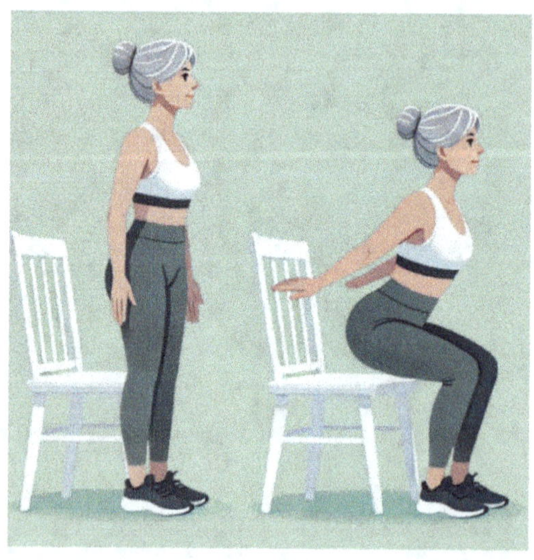

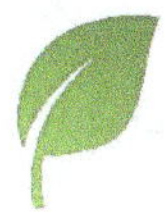

6. Chest Press

- **Steps**:

    1. Lie flat on a bench or mat with a dumbbell in each hand, arms extended above the chest.

    2. Slowly bend your elbows to lower the dumbbells to chest level.

    3. Press the weights back up to the starting position.

    4. Complete 8-10 repetitions.

- **Benefits**: Strengthens the chest, shoulders, and triceps.

- **Variations**: Perform on an incline bench to target different angles of the chest.

- **Safety Tips**: Keep the movement controlled, especially when lowering the weights to avoid straining the shoulder joint.

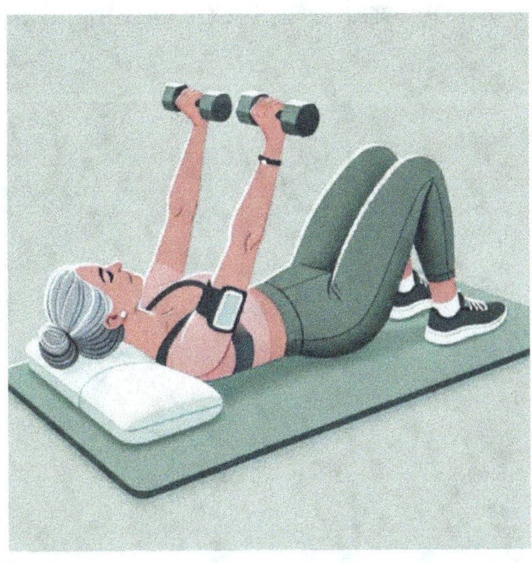

7. Core Twist

- **Steps**:

  1. Sit on the edge of a chair with your feet flat on the floor.

  2. Hold a medicine ball or weight close to your chest.

  3. Rotate your torso to the right, moving the ball to the right side.

  4. Rotate back to the center and then to the left side.

  5. Repeat the sequence 10 times on each side.

- **Benefits**: Strengthens the abdominal and oblique muscles, improves rotational mobility.

- **Variations**: Increase the weight of the ball to intensify the workout.

- **Safety Tips**: Keep your movements slow and controlled to prevent any jerking that could harm the back.

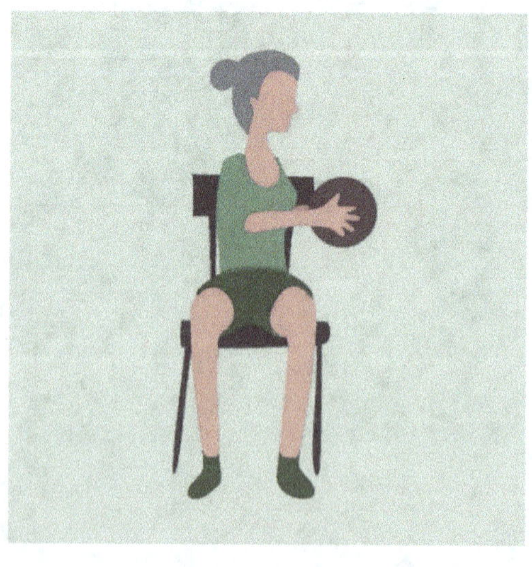

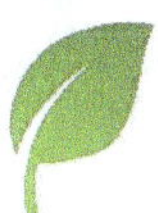

8. Deadlifts

- **Steps**:

    1. Stand with your feet hip-width apart, a dumbbell in front of each foot.

    2. Bend at your hips and knees, keeping your back flat.

    4. Grab the dumbbells with an overhand grip, arms straight.

    5. Lift the dumbbells by straightening your hips and knees.

    6. Lower the dumbbells back to the ground.

    7. Perform 8-12 repetitions.

- **Benefits**: Strengthens the lower back, hamstrings, and glutes.

- **Variations**: Use a barbell for traditional deadlifts or kettlebells for variation.

- **Safety Tips**: Keep your back straight and lift with your legs, not your back, to prevent injury.

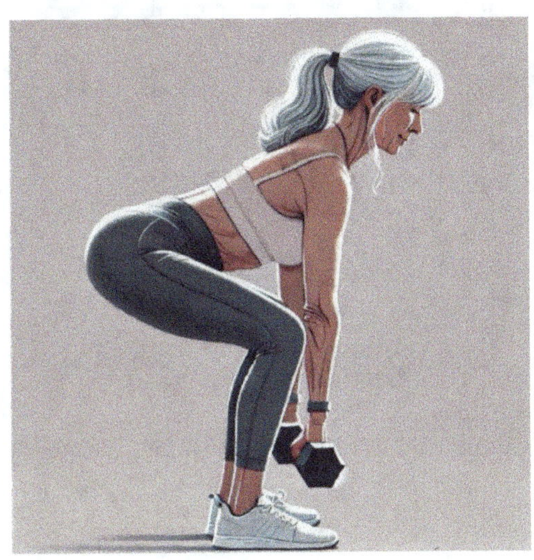

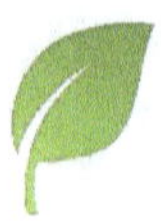

9. Dumbbell Rows

- **Steps**:

  1. Hold a dumbbell in one hand and stand with feet hip-width apart.

  2. Bend slightly at the waist so your torso is almost parallel to the floor.

  3. Pull the dumbbell upward to the side of your chest, keeping the arm close to your side.

  4. Lower the dumbbell slowly back to the starting position.

  5. Perform 10-12 repetitions on each side.

- **Benefits**: Strengthens the upper back, shoulders, and biceps.

- **Variations**: Perform bent-over rows with both arms simultaneously if balance allows.

- **Safety Tips**: Avoid jerking motions; ensure a controlled lift and descent.

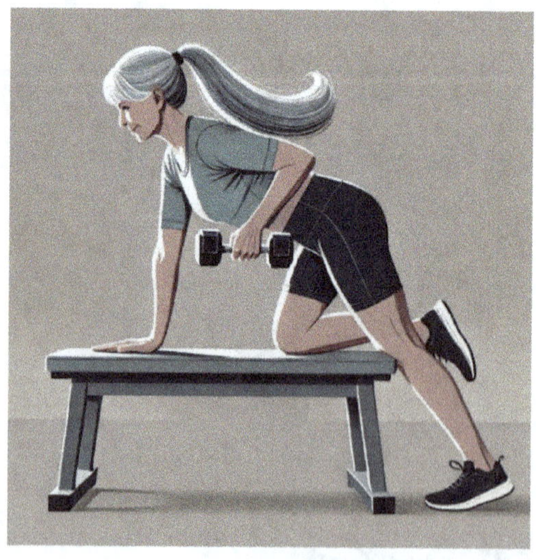

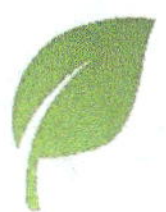

10. Dumbbell Shoulder Press

- **Steps**:

    1. Sit or stand with a dumbbell in each hand at shoulder height, elbows bent.

    2. Press the dumbbells upward until your arms are fully extended above your head.

    3. Lower the dumbbells back to shoulder height.

    4. Perform 8-10 repetitions.

- **Benefits**: Works the shoulders and upper arms.

- **Variations**: Alternate arms or add a twist to engage your core.

- **Safety Tips**: Do not arch your back; maintain a strong, stable posture.

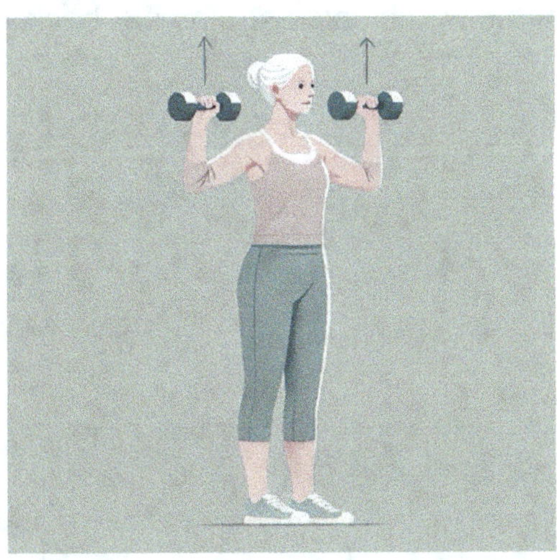

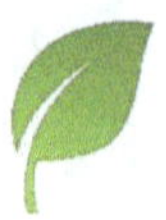

11. Dumbbell Side Bends

- **Steps**:

    1. Stand with your feet hip-width apart, a dumbbell in one hand.

    2. Keep your back straight and shoulders level.

    3. Slowly bend to the side where you hold the dumbbell, feeling a stretch on the opposite side.

    4. Return to the upright position and repeat 10-12 times.

    5. Switch the dumbbell to the other hand and repeat.

- **Benefits**: Strengthens obliques and promotes lateral flexibility.

- **Variations**: Perform without weights as a gentle stretch.

- **Safety Tips**: Move smoothly to avoid any jerking movements which could strain your back.

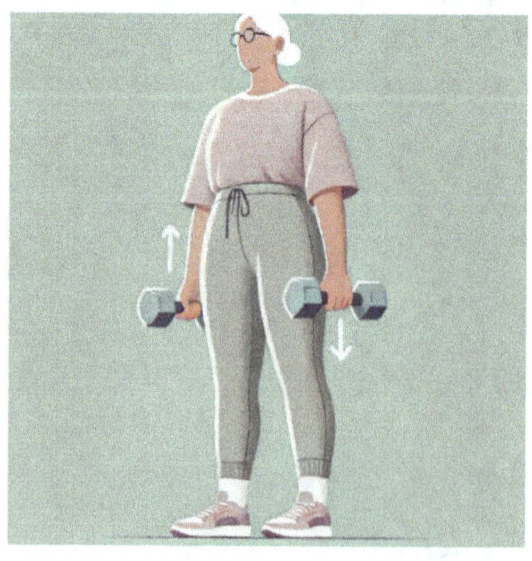

12. Forward Arm Raises

- **Steps**:

  1. Stand or sit with your back straight and a dumbbell in each hand.

  2. With palms facing down, lift the arms straight in front of you to shoulder height.

  3. Lower the arms back down smoothly.

  4. Perform 10-15 repetitions.

- **Benefits**: Strengthens the shoulder muscles, specifically the anterior deltoids.

- **Variations**: Lift one arm at a time to focus on stability.

- **Safety Tips**: Do not swing the dumbbells; lift and lower in a controlled manner to prevent momentum use.

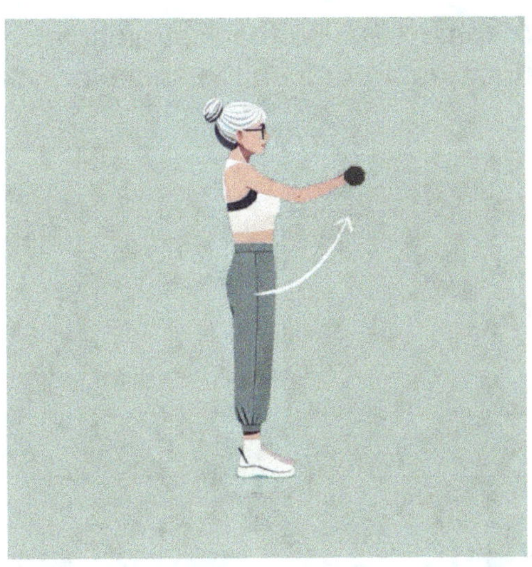

13. Hamstring Stretches

- **Steps**:

    1. Sit on the ground with one leg extended straight in front of you, the other leg bent with the foot flat against the opposite inner thigh.

    2. Lean forward from your hips towards the foot of your extended leg.

    8. Reach your hands toward your toes or as far as you can go without rounding your back.

    9. Hold the stretch for 15-30 seconds, then switch legs and repeat.

- **Benefits**: Increases flexibility in the hamstrings and lower back, which can help prevent back pain.

- **Variations**: Perform the stretch while seated in a chair, extending one leg out on another chair in front of you.

- **Safety Tips**: Keep your back straight and bend from the hips rather than rounding the spine to avoid strain.

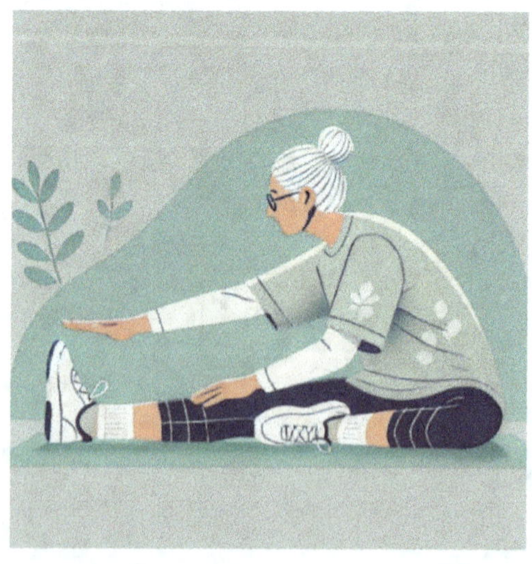

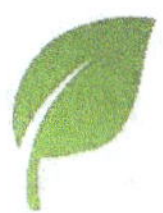

14. Heel-to-Toe Walk

- **Steps**:

  1. Stand upright and place the heel of one foot just in front of the toes of the opposite foot each time you take a step.

  2. Focus on a point in the distance to maintain balance.

  3. Walk 20 steps in a heel-to-toe manner.

- **Benefits**: Improves balance and coordination, essential for preventing falls.

- **Variations**: Perform the exercise along a straight line or use a wall or a chair for balance support if needed.

- **Safety Tips**: Start this exercise near a wall or with a chair close by to grab onto if you feel unsteady.

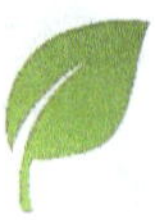

15. High Knees

- **Steps**:

    1. Stand with your feet hip-width apart.

    2. Lift one knee to the chest, then quickly switch to lift the opposite knee.

    3. Continue to alternate knees, pumping your arms in coordination with your legs.

    4. Perform this movement for 30 seconds to 1 minute.

- **Benefits**: Enhances lower body strength, cardiovascular health, and coordination.

- **Variations**: Slow down the pace to reduce intensity or if you're new to the exercise.

- **Safety Tips**: If balancing is difficult, perform the exercise while holding onto a stable surface.

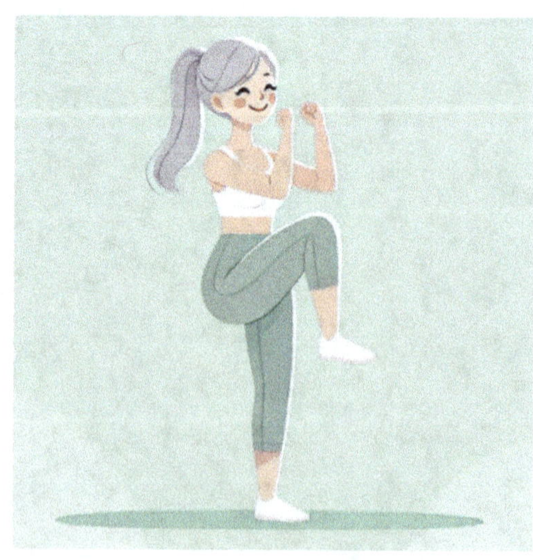

16. Hip Flexor Stretch

- **Steps**:

  1. Kneel on one knee, with the other foot in front, foot flat on the floor and knee bent at a 90-degree angle.

  2. Push your hips forward gently until you feel a stretch in the upper thigh of your back leg.

  3. Hold the stretch for 20-30 seconds, then switch legs and repeat.

- **Benefits**: Loosens hip flexor muscles, which can help alleviate lower back pain and improve posture.

- **Variations**: For a deeper stretch, raise the arm (on the same side as the back leg) over your head while leaning slightly forward.

- **Safety Tips**: Keep the body straight and avoid leaning too far forward, which could strain the lower back.

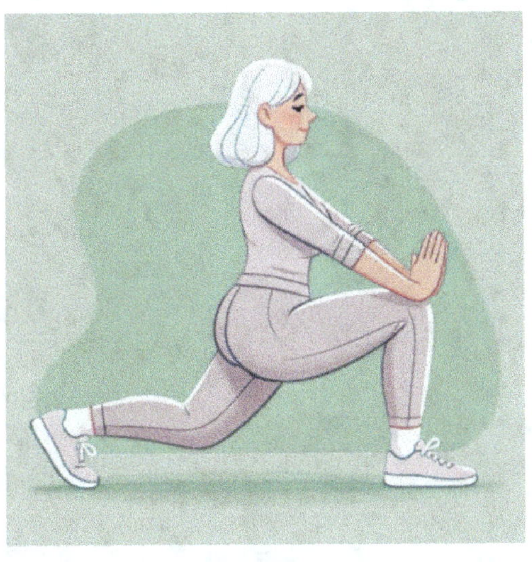

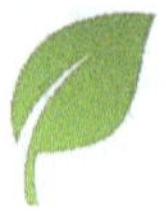

17. Knee Lifts

- **Steps**:

    1. Stand with your feet hip-width apart and arms at your sides or on your hips for balance.

    2. Slowly lift one knee towards your chest as high as comfortably possible.

    3. Lower the knee and repeat with the other leg.

    4. Alternate legs for 10-15 repetitions on each side.

- **Benefits**: Strengthens the lower abdominals and hip flexors, enhances balance and coordination.

- **Variations**: Add ankle weights for increased resistance.

- **Safety Tips**: Perform the exercise near a chair or counter to hold onto if you need extra support.

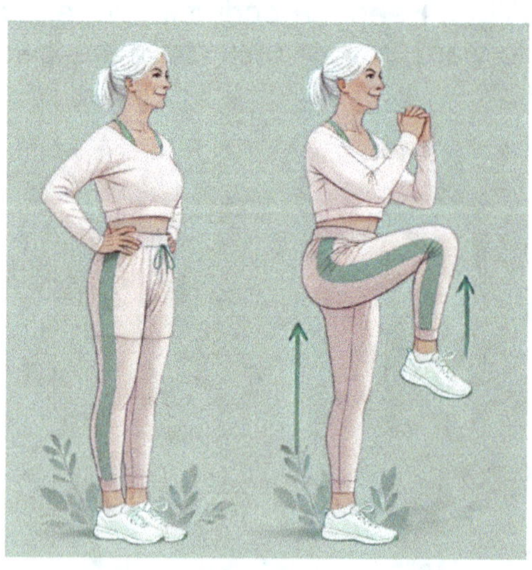

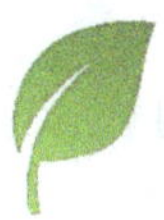

18. Leg Lifts

- **Steps**:

    1. Lie on your side with your legs straight and stacked on top of each other.

    2. Prop your head up with your hand or rest it on your arm.

    3. Lift the top leg upwards while keeping it straight, then lower it back down.

    4. Perform 10-15 repetitions, then switch to the other side and repeat.

- **Benefits**: Strengthens the hip abductors and stabilizes the hips.

- **Variations**: Perform the lifts with a resistance band around your thighs to increase difficulty.

- **Safety Tips**: Keep movements controlled to avoid jerking, which could cause muscle strain.

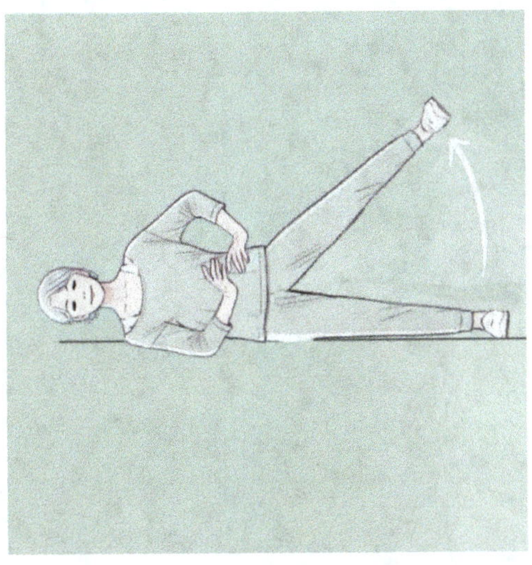

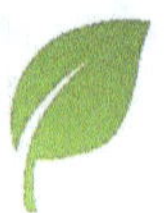

19. Leg Stretches

- **Steps**:

  1. Sit on the floor with your legs extended straight in front of you.

  2. Reach forward towards your toes with both hands, keeping your knees straight.

  3. Hold the stretch for 15-30 seconds, feeling a stretch along the back of your legs.

- **Benefits**: Increases flexibility in the hamstrings and lower back, promoting better posture and reducing the risk of back pain.

- **Variations**: If reaching for your toes is difficult, use a towel or yoga strap to help pull yourself forward.

- **Safety Tips**: Bend from the hips and keep your back straight to prevent unnecessary strain.

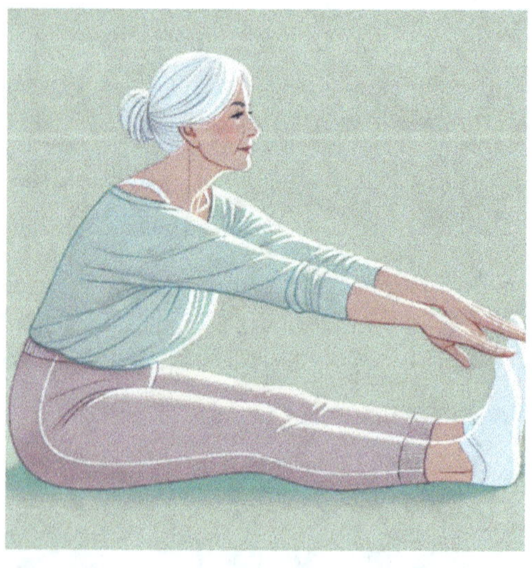

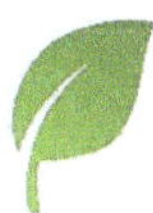

20. Lunge and Twist

- **Steps**:

    1. Stand with your feet together and take a large step forward with one leg.

    2. Lower your hips until both knees are bent at about a 90-degree angle.

    3. Place your opposite hand to your forward leg on your thigh, and twist your torso towards the forward leg.

    4. Hold the twist for a few seconds, then return to the starting position and switch legs.

- **Benefits**: Enhances leg strength, flexibility, and core stability; the twist helps improve spinal mobility.

- **Variations**: Hold a medicine ball in front of your chest to add a dynamic challenge to the twist.

- **Safety Tips**: Keep your forward knee directly above your ankle and not pushed too far forward to protect the knee joint.

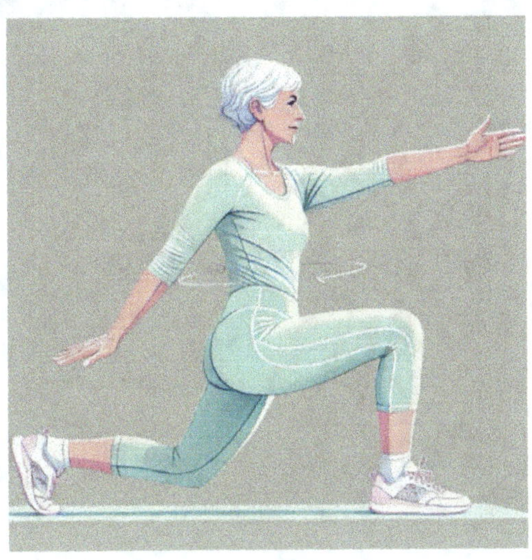

21. Neck Rolls

- **Steps**:

    1.   Sit or stand with your back straight and shoulders relaxed.

    2.   Drop your chin towards your chest, then slowly roll your head to one side, back, and around to the other side.

    4.   Repeat the motion several times in each direction.

- **Benefits**: Relieves tension in the neck and upper shoulders.

- **Variations**: Vary the speed and range of the rolls based on your comfort level.

- **Safety Tips**: Move slowly and smoothly to avoid straining the neck muscles.

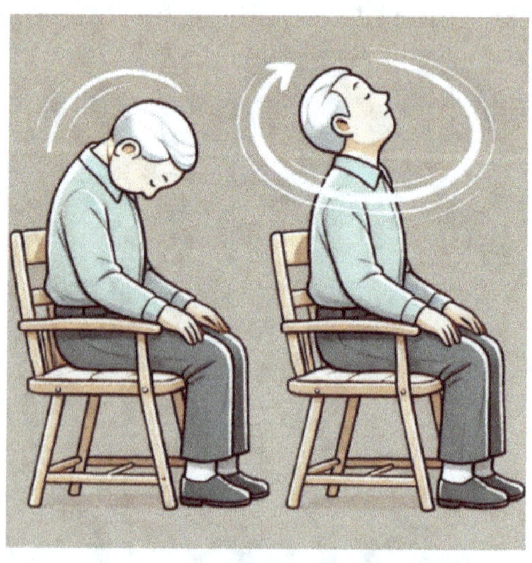

22. Overhead Arm Raises

- **Steps**:

    1. Sit or stand with your arms at your sides and a dumbbell in each hand.

    2. Slowly raise your arms straight above your head.

    3. Lower them back down to your sides.

    4. Repeat for 10-15 repetitions.

- **Benefits**: Strengthens the shoulders and upper arms, improves range of motion in the shoulders.

- **Variations**: Perform one arm at a time to focus on unilateral strength.

- **Safety Tips**: Keep the weights appropriate to your strength level to avoid overexertion.

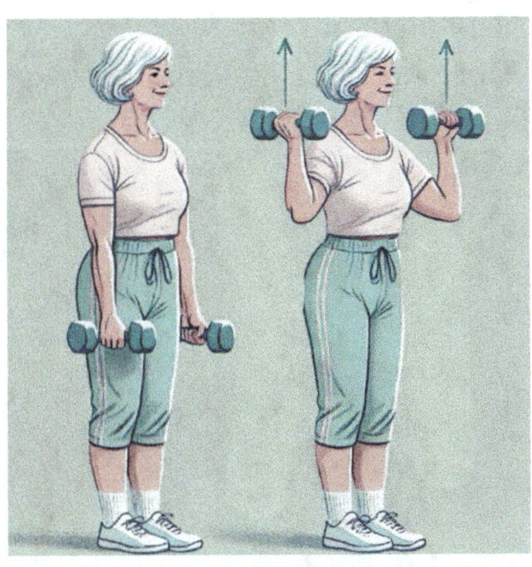

23. Plank Holds

- **Steps**:

    1. Start in a push-up position but bend your elbows and rest your weight on your forearms instead of your hands.

    2. Ensure your body forms a straight line from your shoulders to your ankles.

    5. Engage your core by sucking your belly button into your spine.

    6. Hold this position for 20-30 seconds or as long as you can maintain proper form.

- **Benefits**: Strengthens the core, shoulders, and hips, and improves balance and posture.

- **Variations**: Perform a side plank to focus on the oblique muscles or a knee plank if you need a less intense option.

- **Safety Tips**: Avoid letting your hips sag or lifting them too high, as this can strain your back.

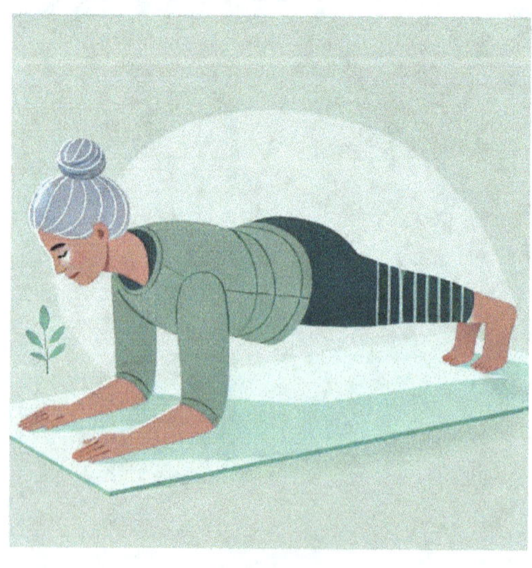

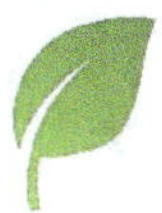

24. Seated Forward Bend

- **Steps**:

    1. Sit on a chair with your feet flat on the floor.

    2. Keep your back straight, inhale and raise your arms above your head.

    3. As you exhale, bend forward at the hips and lower your arms towards your toes.

    4. Reach as far as comfortable, then hold the position for a few seconds.

    5. Slowly sit back up to the starting position.

- **Benefits**: Stretches the spine and hamstrings; promotes flexibility in the lower back.

- **Variations**: Extend one leg at a time for a deeper hamstring stretch.

- **Safety Tips**: Bend from the hips, not the waist, and do not force the bend beyond your comfort level.

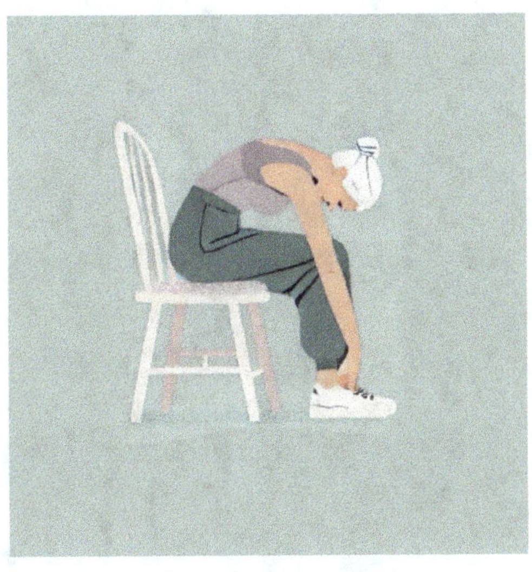

25. Seated Hamstring Stretch

- **Steps**:

  1. Sit on the edge of a chair and extend one leg out with the heel on the floor and the toe pointing up.

  2. Sit up straight, then lean forward from your hips towards the extended leg.

  3. Hold the stretch for 20-30 seconds, feeling a pull along the back of your thigh.

  4. Repeat on the other leg.

- **Benefits**: Improves flexibility in the hamstrings, which can reduce lower back discomfort.

- **Variations**: Use a towel or strap around your foot to pull gently if you cannot reach your toes.

- **Safety Tips**: Keep your back straight as you lean forward to prevent rounding, which can strain the back.

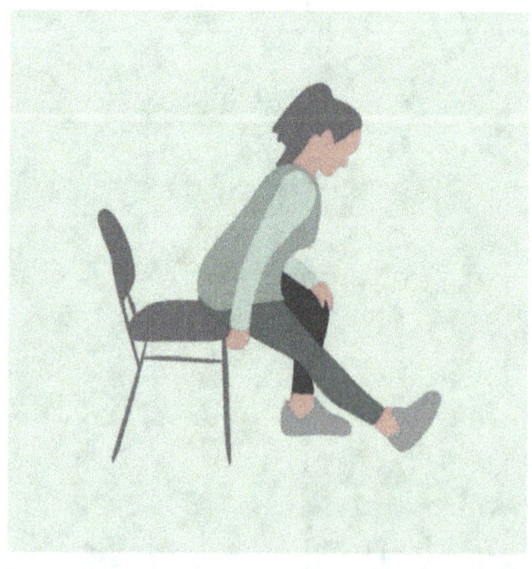

26. Seated Leg Extensions

- **Steps**:

  1. Sit in a chair with your feet flat on the floor.

  3. Slowly extend one leg until it is horizontal and hold for a few seconds.

  4. Lower the leg back down without letting it touch the floor and repeat.

  5. Perform 10-15 repetitions on each leg.

- **Benefits**: Strengthens the quadriceps, which are important for knee stability and mobility.

- **Variations**: Add ankle weights to increase resistance.

- **Safety Tips**: Move in a controlled manner to avoid jerking, which could strain the knee.

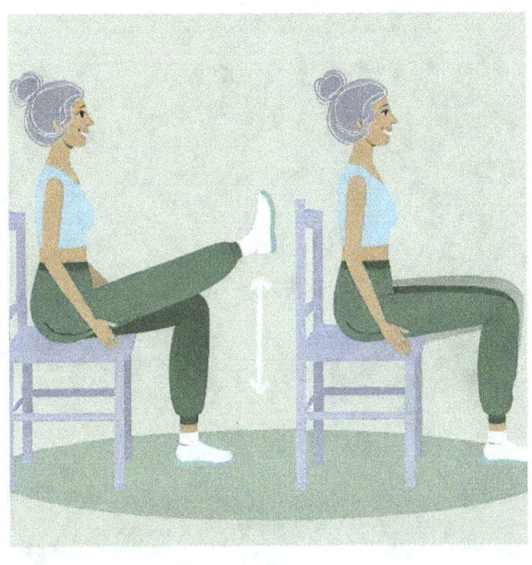

27. Seated Side Stretch

- **Steps**:

  1. Sit upright in a chair, feet flat on the floor.

  2. Raise one arm over your head and lean to the opposite side, bending at the waist.

  3. Hold the stretch for 10-15 seconds, feeling a stretch along your side.

  4. Return to the starting position and repeat on the other side.

- **Benefits**: Enhances lateral flexibility of the spine and stretches the muscles of the side torso.

- **Variations**: Hold a light weight in the raised hand to deepen the stretch.

- **Safety Tips**: Keep your movements gentle and controlled; do not overextend to avoid strain on the side muscles and spine.

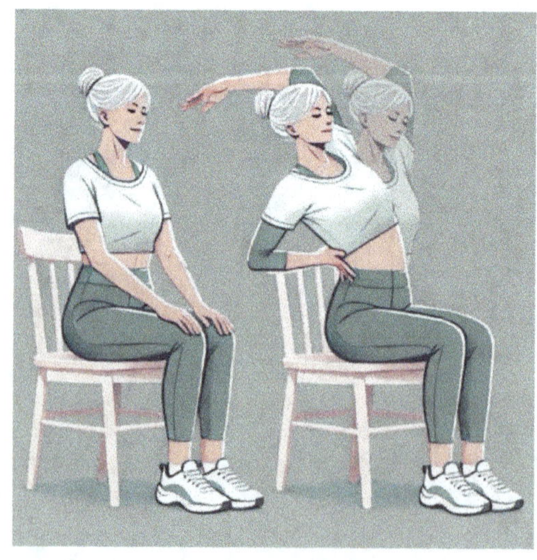

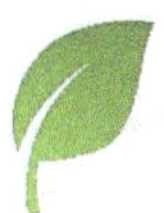

28. Seated Spinal Twist

- **Steps**:

  1. Sit upright in a chair with your feet flat on the floor.

  2. Place your right hand on the back of the chair and your left hand on your right knee.

  3. Gently twist your torso to the right, using your arms to deepen the twist.

  5. Hold the position for 10-15 seconds, then slowly return to the starting position.

  6. Repeat on the opposite side.

- **Benefits**: Improves spinal mobility and can help alleviate back pain. It also aids in digestion.

- **Variations**: Deepen the twist by looking over your shoulder in the direction of the twist.

- **Safety Tips**: Twist only as far as comfortable; avoid forcing the twist to prevent back strain.

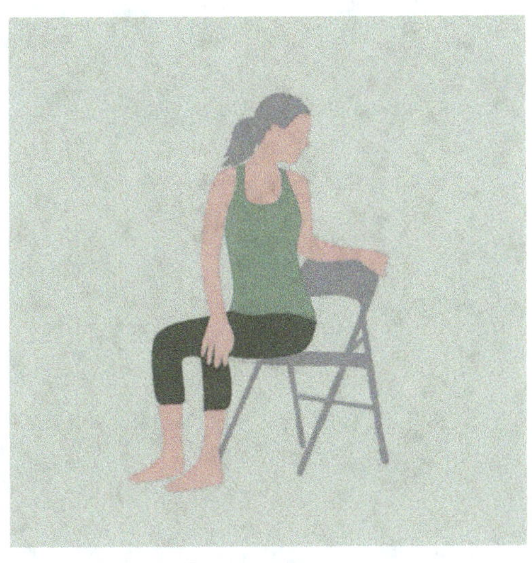

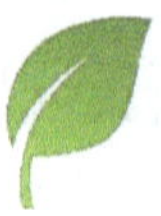

29. Seated Toe Taps

- **Steps**:

  1. Sit in a chair with your feet flat on the floor and back straight.

  2. Lift the toes of one foot while keeping your heel on the ground, then tap the toes back down.

  3. Alternate feet, performing the movement for 10-15 repetitions per foot.

- **Benefits**: Strengthens the muscles in the lower legs and improves ankle mobility.

- **Variations**: Increase speed or add ankle weights for more challenge.

- **Safety Tips**: Perform the movement in a controlled manner to avoid jerking the leg.

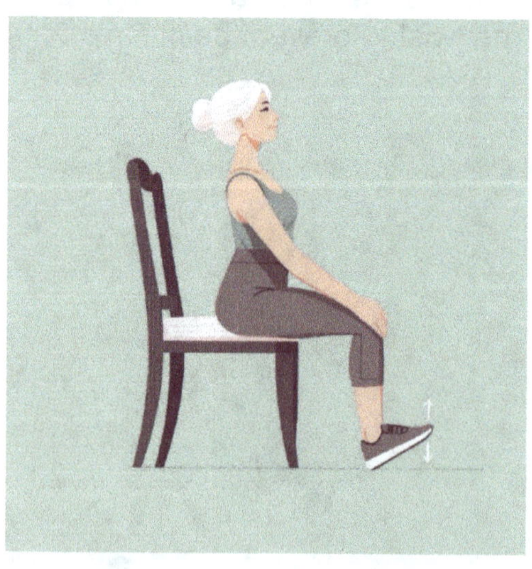

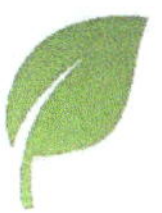

30. Shoulder Press

- **Steps**:

    1. Stand or sit with hands at shoulder height, elbows bent and palms facing forward.

    2. Press the weights upward until your arms are fully extended above your head.

    3. Pause briefly at the top, then slowly lower the hands back to shoulder height.

    4. Repeat for 8-12 repetitions.

- **Benefits**: Strengthens the shoulder muscles, upper back, and arms.

- **Variations**: Perform the exercise seated for stability, especially if standing balance is a concern.

- **Safety Tips**: Ensure not to arch your back as you press the weights; keep your core engaged.

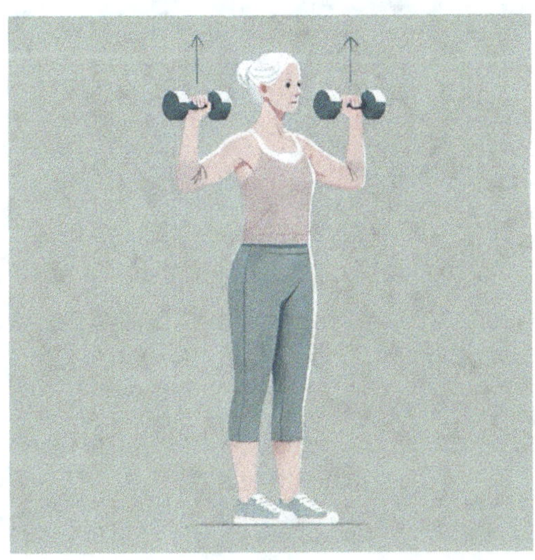

31. Shoulder Rolls

- **Steps**:

    1. Sit or stand with your back straight and arms relaxed at your sides.

    2. Slowly roll your shoulders up towards your ears, then back, and down in a circular motion.

    3. Perform 10-15 rolls in each direction.

- **Benefits**: Reduces tension in the shoulder and neck area, promotes relaxation.

- **Variations**: Increase the range of motion to intensify the stretch.

- **Safety Tips**: Perform the rolls slowly to avoid creating tension in the neck.

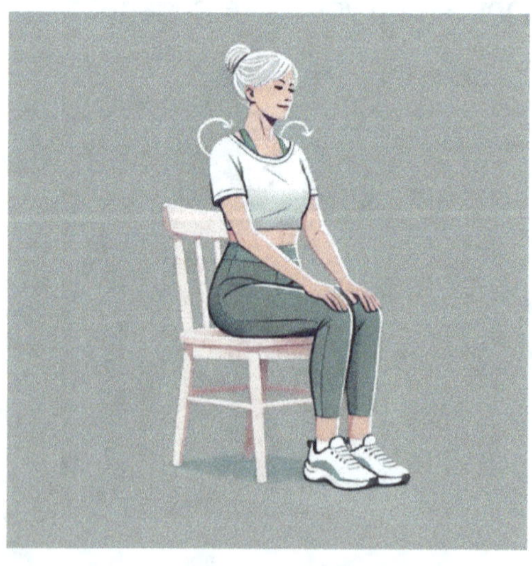

32. Side Leg Raises

- **Steps**:

  1. Stand beside a chair or counter for support.

  2. Slowly lift one leg to the side, keeping it straight, then lower it back down.

  3. Perform 10-15 repetitions, then switch to the other leg.

- **Benefits**: Strengthens the hip abductors, which are crucial for maintaining balance and stability.

- **Variations**: Add ankle weights to increase resistance.

- **Safety Tips**: Keep your body upright and avoid leaning to the opposite side as you lift your leg.

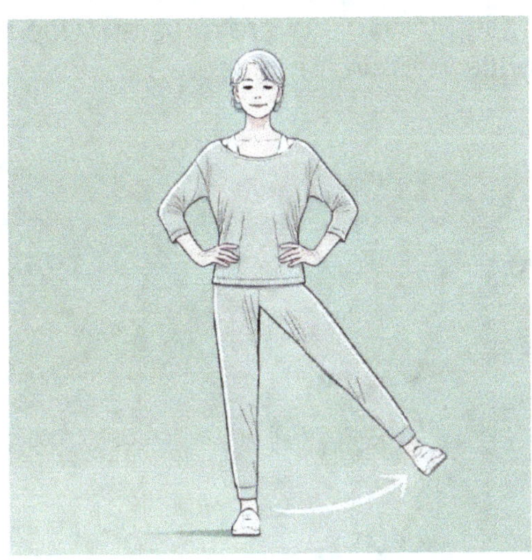

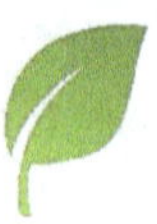

33. Single-Leg Deadlifts

- **Steps**:

    1. Stand on one leg, holding a dumbbell in the opposite hand.

    6. Bend forward at the hip, extending the free leg behind you for balance, and lower the dumbbell towards the floor.

    7. Slowly return to the starting position, keeping your balance throughout the movement.

    8. Perform 8-10 repetitions on each side.

- **Benefits**: Enhances balance, strengthens the glutes, hamstrings, and lower back.

- **Variations**: Perform without weights until you're comfortable with the balance aspects.

- **Safety Tips**: Keep a slight bend in the knee of the standing leg to avoid overextension. Use a wall or chair for balance support if needed.

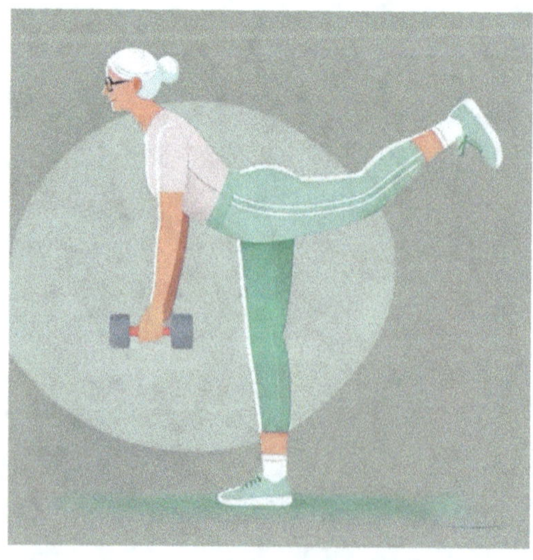

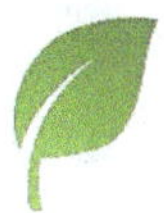

34. Standing Quadricep Stretch

- **Steps**:

    1. Stand on one leg, using a chair for balance.

    2. Bend your free leg, bringing your heel towards your buttock, and grasp your ankle with your hand.

    9. Hold the stretch for 15-30 seconds, feeling a stretch in the front of your thigh.

    10. Repeat on the other leg.

- **Benefits**: Stretches the quadriceps, which ations**: If you cannot reach your ankle, use a towel or resistance band to help pull the heel closer.

- **Safety Tips**: Maintain good posture by keeping your knees close together and your torso upright. Avoid pulling excessively on the foot if you feel any knee discomfort.

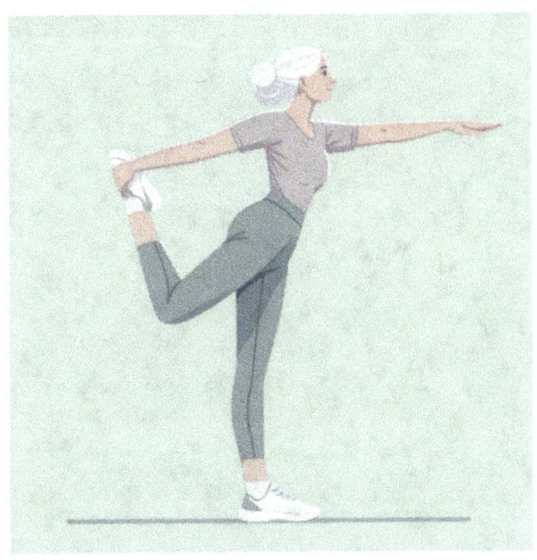

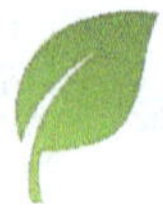

35. Step-Ups

- **Steps**:

  1. Stand in front of a sturdy step or platform.

  2. Step up with one foot, pressing through your heel to bring your other foot up onto the step.

  3. Step down with the leading foot, followed by the trailing foot, to return to the starting position.

  4. Alternate the leading leg with each set or after several repetitions.

- **Benefits**: Builds strength in the legs, particularly the thighs and glutes; enhances coordination and balance.

- **Variations**: Increase the height of the step or add weights to increase difficulty.

- **Safety Tips**: Ensure the step is stable and at a suitable height to prevent strain on the knees. Use a handrail if available for balance.

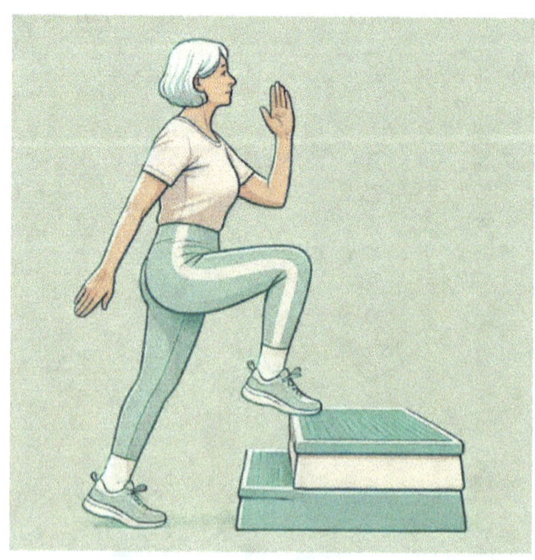

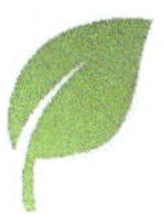

36. Tricep Extensions

- **Steps**:

  1. Stand or sit with a dumbbell held by both hands. Extend your arms over your head.

  2. Keeping your elbows close to your head, slowly bend your elbows to lower the dumbbell behind your head.

  3. Extend your arms back to the starting position.

- **Benefits**: Strengthens the triceps, important for upper body strength and functional movements like pushing.

- **Variations**: Perform one arm at a time with a single dumbbell for increased focus on each tricep.

- **Safety Tips**: Keep your elbows stationary throughout the exercise and move only your forearms. Avoid using excessive weight, which can lead to poor form and potential injury.

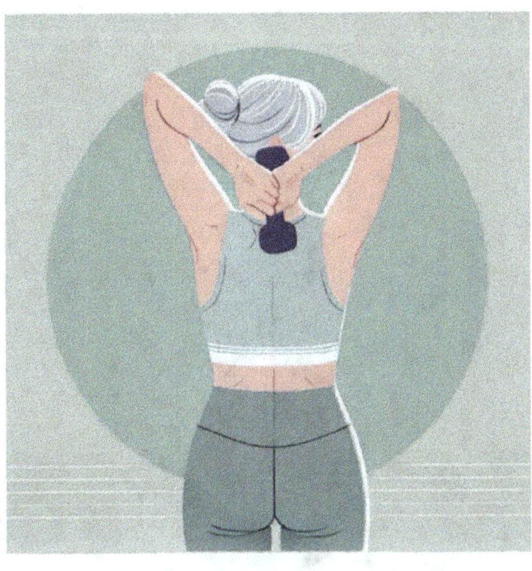

37. Wall Push-Ups

- **Steps**:

  1. Face a wall, standing a little farther than arm's length away, feet shoulder-width apart.

  2. Place your palms against the wall at shoulder height and shoulder-width apart.

  3. Bend your elbows and lean your body toward the wall.

  4. Push yourself back to the starting position.

- **Benefits**: Strengthens the chest, shoulders, and arms with less strain on the wrists and back than floor push-ups.

- **Variations**: Adjust the distance of your feet from the wall to increase or decrease resistance.

- **Safety Tips**: Ensure your body is in a straight line from head to heels and that you engage your core to prevent sagging of the hips.

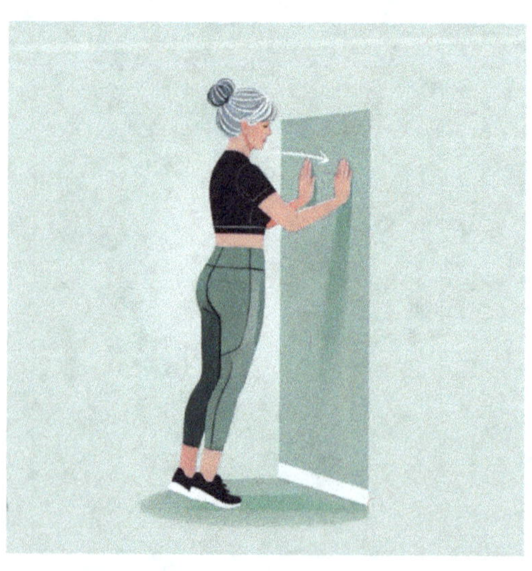

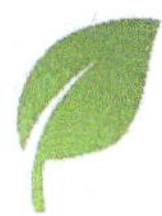

38. Water Aerobics

- **Steps**:

  1. Join a class or follow a water aerobics routine in a pool.

  2. Perform aerobic exercises that are typically done on land, such as walking, jumping jacks, and arm circles, adapted for water resistance.

- **Benefits**: Provides buoyancy that reduces stress on joints, muscles, and bones while offering resistance training.

- **Variations**: Use water weights or noodles to increase resistance and intensity.

- **Safety Tips**: Always perform water aerobics in a safe depth and consider wearing water shoes to prevent slipping.

CHAIR YOGA EXERCISES

39. Chair Cat-Cow Stretch

- **Steps**:

    1. Sit in a chair with your feet flat on the floor, hands on your knees.

    2. Inhale, arch your back and tilt your head and shoulders back (Cow position).

    3. Exhale, round your spine, tucking your chin to your chest and pulling your belly in (Cat position).

    4. Continue flowing smoothly between Cow and Cat for several breaths.

- **Benefits**: Increases flexibility and mobility in the spine, relieves tension in the back and neck.

- **Variations**: Intensify the stretch by increasing the range of motion.

- **Safety Tips**: Move gently between the positions without forcing the spine beyond its comfortable range of motion.

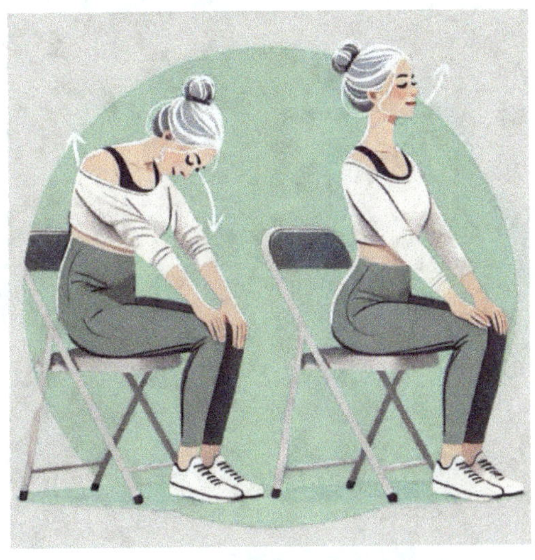

40. Chair Forward Bend

- **Steps**:

  1. Sit on the edge of a chair with your feet wider than hip-width apart.

  2. Exhale and slowly bend forward, lowering your torso between your legs.

  4. Allow your hands to rest on the floor or hold onto your ankles.

  5. Hold the position for a few breaths, then slowly rise back to a seated position.

- **Benefits**: Stretches the back and hamstrings, promotes relaxation.

- **Variations**: For a deeper stretch, extend your arms forward on the floor.

- **Safety Tips**: Bend from the hips and not the waist to keep the spine aligned and prevent strain.

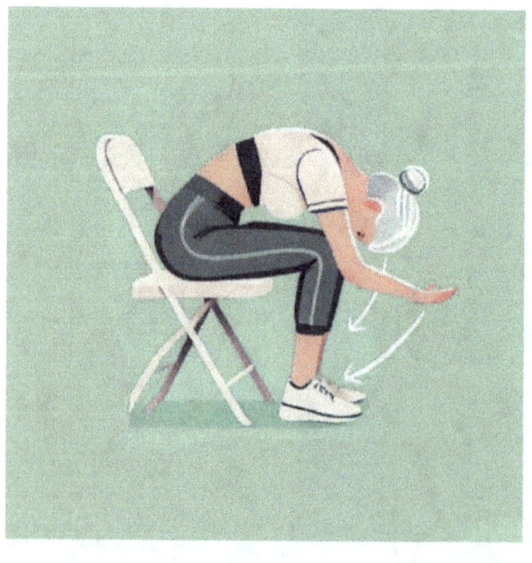

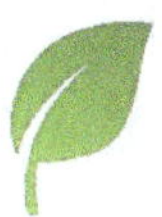

41. Chair Extended Side Angle

- **Steps**:

    1. Sit sideways on a chair, legs extended to one side, and feet flat.

    2. Extend the arm on the side of the chair upward, reaching over your head while you gently lean your torso over the chair.

    3. Hold the position for a few breaths, then switch sides and repeat.

- **Benefits**: Stretches the sides of the body, enhances lateral flexibility, improves balance.

- **Variations**: Adjust the stretch by modifying the reach of the arm.

- **Safety Tips**: Keep your seated posture upright and stable; avoid leaning too far to prevent falling off the chair.

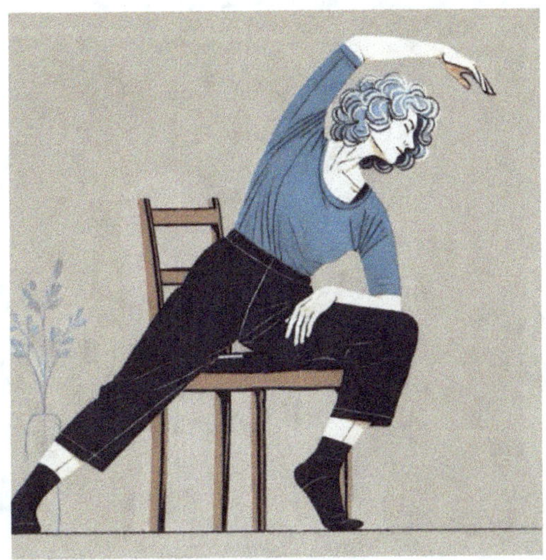

42. Chair Pigeon

- **Steps**:

    1. While seated, place your right ankle on your left thigh just above the knee.

    2. Keep your back straight and gently lean forward to intensify the stretch.

    6. Hold this position for several breaths, then switch legs and repeat.

- **Benefits**: Opens up the hips, stretches the thighs and glutes.

- **Variations**: Adjust the depth of the forward lean to increase or decrease the stretch intensity.

- **Safety Tips**: Ensure you do not feel pain in your knee; adjust your foot and ankle positioning if necessary.

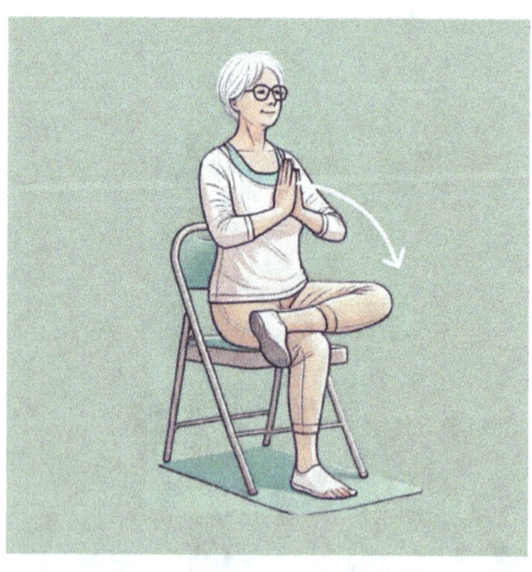

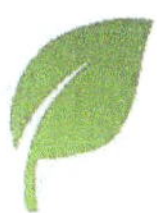

43. Chair Warrior I

- **Steps**:

  1. Sit sideways on a chair, one leg bent with the foot flat on the floor, and the other leg extended back, resting on the toes.

  3. Raise your arms above your head, palms facing each other.

  4. Hold the pose while gently turning your torso toward the bent knee.

  5. Maintain the pose for several breaths, then switch sides and repeat.

- **Benefits**: Strengthens the legs, improves focus, stretches the arms and back.

- **Variations**: For less intensity, keep your arms at chest level or placed on your hips.

- **Safety Tips**: Ensure the chair is stable and avoid overstretching, especially in the back leg.

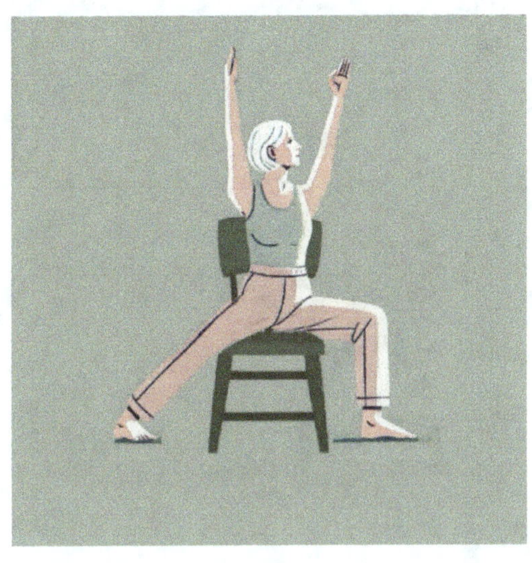

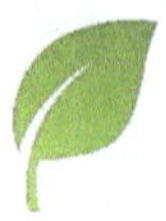

44. Chair Tree Pose

- **Steps**:

    1. Sit with your back straight and feet flat on the floor.

    2. Place the sole of your right foot on the inside of your left thigh, keeping your right knee bent to the side.

    3. Bring your hands together in a prayer position at your chest.

    5. Hold the pose for several breaths, then switch sides and repeat.

- **Benefits**: Improves balance, strengthens thighs, calves, ankles, and spine.

- **Variations**: If placing the foot on the thigh is uncomfortable, position it lower on the leg, but not directly on the knee.

- **Safety Tips**: Focus on a fixed point to maintain balance, and use the back of the chair for support if needed.

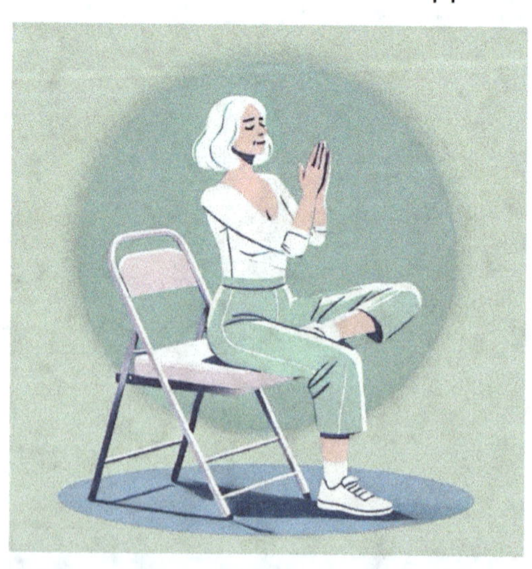

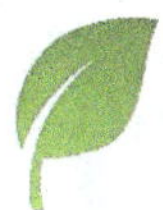

45. Seated Eagle Pose

- **Steps**:

  1. Sit upright in a chair with your feet flat on the floor.

  2. Cross your right thigh over your left thigh as high as you can. If possible, tuck the right foot behind the left calf.

  7. Extend your arms straight in front of your body, then cross the left arm over the right at the elbows. Bend the elbows and try to bring your palms to touch.

  8. Hold the pose for several breaths, focusing on your balance and the stretch in your shoulders and upper back, then switch sides and repeat.

- **Benefits**: Improves focus, balance, and stretches the shoulders, arms, hips, and legs.

- **Variations**: If the full arm wrap is too challenging, simply press the backs of the hands together.

- **Safety Tips**: Ensure you maintain even breathing and do not strain any joints, particularly the knees and wrists.

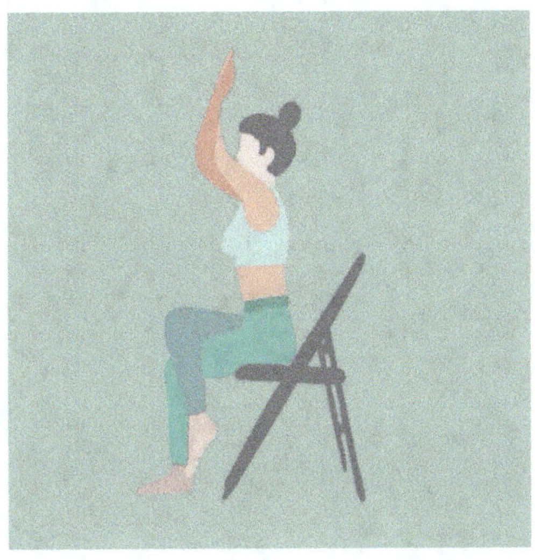

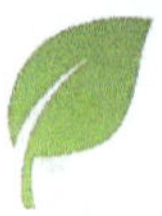

46. Seated Mountain Pose

- **Steps**:

  1. Sit at the front edge of a chair with your feet flat on the floor, hip-width apart.

  2. Extend your spine, lifting through the crown of your head to sit as tall as possible.

  3. Relax your shoulders down away from your ears, and place your hands on your thighs or along your sides.

  4. Breathe deeply, feeling your torso rise and fall with each breath. Hold the pose for 30 seconds to one minute.

- **Benefits**: Promotes good posture, enhances focus, and provides a foundation for other seated exercises.

- **Variations**: Raise your arms overhead for an added stretch through the torso.

- **Safety Tips**: Keep your chin level and gaze straight ahead to maintain a neutral neck position.

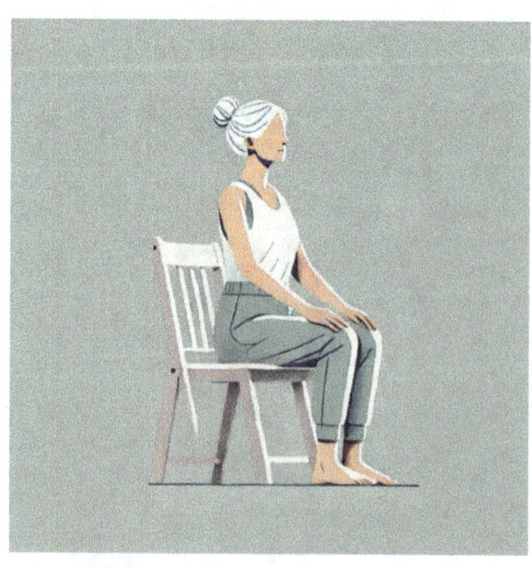